LONDON MATHEMATICAL SOCIETY LECTURE NC

Managing Editor: Professor M. Reid, Mathematics Institute,
University of Warwick, Coventry CV4 7AL, United Kingdom

The titles below are available from booksellers, or from Cambridge University Press at www.cambridge.org/mathematics

London Mathematical Society Lecture Note Series: 369

Epidemics and Rumours in Complex Networks

MOEZ DRAIEF
Imperial College, London

LAURENT MASSOULIÉ
Thomson Corporate Research, Paris

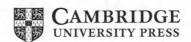
CAMBRIDGE
UNIVERSITY PRESS

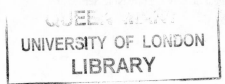
CAMBRIDGE UNIVERSITY PRESS
Cambridge, New York, Melbourne, Madrid, Cape Town, Singapore, São Paulo, Delhi

Cambridge University Press
The Edinburgh Building, Cambridge CB2 8RU, UK

Published in the United States of America by Cambridge University Press, New York

www.cambridge.org
Information on this title: www.cambridge.org/9780521734431

© M. Draief and L. Massoulié 2010

First published 2010

Printed in the United Kingdom at the University Press, Cambridge

A catalogue record for this publication is available from the British Library

Library of Congress Cataloguing in Publication data
Draief, Moez, 1978–
Epidemics and rumours in complex networks / Moez Draief, Laurent Massoulié.
p.   cm. – (London Mathematical Society lecture note series ; 369)
Includes bibliographical references and index.
ISBN 978-0-521-73443-1 (pbk.)
1. Computer security – Mathematics.   2. Epidemics – Computer simulation.
3. Biologically-inspired computing.   4. Graph theory.   5. Probabilities.
I. Massoulié, Laurent.   II. Title.   III. Series.
QA76.9.A25D78   2010
004.6 – dc22   2009032956

ISBN 978-0-521-73443-1 Paperback

Contents

Introduction

The idea of mimicking the propagation of biological epidemics to achieve diffusion of useful information was first proposed in the late 1980s, the decade that also saw the appearance of computer viruses. Back then, these viruses propagated by copies on floppy disks and caused much less harm than their contemporary versions. But it was already noticed that they evolved and survived much as biological viruses do, a fact that prompted the idea of putting these features to good (rather than evil) use. The first application to be considered was synchronisation of distributed databases.

Interest in this paradigm received new impetus with the advent of peer-to-peer systems, online social systems and wireless mobile ad hoc networks in the early 2000s. All these scenarios feature a complex network with potentially evolving connections. In such large-scale dynamic environments, epidemic diffusion of information is especially appealing: it is decentralised, and it relies on randomised decisions which can prove as efficient as carefully made decisions. Detailed accounts of epidemic algorithms can be found in papers by Birman *et al.* [12] and Eugster *et al.* [33]. Their applications are manifold. They can be used to perform distributed computation of global statistics in a spatially extended environment (e.g. mean temperature seen by a collection of sensors), to perform real-time delivery of video data streams (e.g. to users receiving live TV via peer-to-peer systems over the internet) and to propagate updates of dynamic content (e.g. to mobile phone users whose phone operating system requires patching against vulnerabilities).

This book is meant as an introduction for applied mathematicians and computer scientists to the study of epidemic propagation over complex networks. The book's first purpose is to provide the reader with an accessible introduction to the elementary models of epidemic propagation, and develop an understanding of the basic *phase transition* phenomena (also called *threshold* phenomena) that are typical of epidemic behaviour. To this end it introduces the relevant generic models, analytical tools, and mathematical results. This book also aims to explain the role played by network topology in the propagation of information.

This book can be used both to accompany courses for graduate students in computer science and applied probability and to provide an overview of the probabilistic techniques widely used to study random processes on complex networks. It evolved from a graduate course given by the authors at Cambridge University from 2005 to 2007. The mathematical prerequisites are reasonable maturity in probability theory at undergraduate level. The main tools introduced in the text consist of large deviations inequalities, coupling of stochastic processes and Poisson approximation.

Readers who want to delve deeper will find thorough treatments of random graphs in Bollobás [13] and Janson *et al.* [42]. The recent book by Durrett [28] also expands on some of the material here, in several directions, in particular on the behaviour of random walks on graphs. Andersson and Britton [3] deals with epidemic modelling in the biological context. Specific suggestions for further reading are also provided at the end of each chapter.

A tour of the book

The text is divided into two distinct but related parts: *shapeless networks* and *structured networks*. The first part (Chapters 1–5) presents techniques for analysing "homogeneous mixing" epidemic processes. In this setting the large population in which the disease spreads has no particular (or totally random, symmetric) topological structure; that is, each individual is the "neighbour" of every other individual. The infection can therefore spread from any infected individual to any healthy one. In particular, this part of the book introduces branching processes, Erdős–Rényi random graphs and so-called Reed–Frost epidemics. Issues such as ultimate outreach and time to global infection are considered.

The second part (Chapters 6–9) covers recent results on the spread of epidemics in structured networks wherein individuals interact with a limited set of neighbours, and where the corresponding topology can exhibit rich structure. It introduces models of such topologically structured networks, including power-law random graphs and navigable small-world graphs. It gives explanatory models for the emergence of such structures, and addresses the impact of structure on the behaviour of epidemics. It also touches upon the algorithmic issue of maximising outbreak as a function of the initial infectives. In what follows we describe the content of the book in more detail and give some perspective on the relevance of each topic to the analysis of epidemic processes on networks.

Chapter 1 reviews elementary results on the Galton–Watson branching process. Branching processes arise naturally in the study of epidemics, as they provide an accurate description of epidemic behaviour in large, shapeless populations, at least in the early stages of dissemination. They are arguably the simplest class of model that exhibits a *phase transition*: the phenomenon by which an infinitesimal variation of microscopic characteristics (here, the offspring distribution) can lead to a macroscopic change in system behaviour (here, infinite survival of the epidemic).

The results of Chapter 1 are then exploited to establish a similar phase transition in a classical epidemic model, namely the Reed–Frost model. In particular, Chapters 2–4 exploit a parallel between the Reed–Frost epidemic model and Erdős–Rényi random graphs to gain insight into the behaviour of the former. Chapter 2 describes a phase transition appearing in the fraction of ultimately infected individuals. Chapter 3 identifies under which parameter ranges an epidemic starting from one infected individual eventually spreads to the whole population. In Chapter 4 we derive an upper bound on the time needed for the epidemic to reach the whole population. Chapter 5 describes a setting in which the microscopic behaviour of the epidemic (how it spreads randomly in the population) can be approximated by a set of differential equations describing the macroscopic or mean-field dynamics of the system. It also introduces some classical models of epidemic spread.

The chapters of the second part of the book cover more advanced topics. These use some techniques introduced in the first part, in particular large deviations inequalities, but are otherwise largely self-contained. Chapter 6 proposes two models and corresponding analyses of the small-world phenomenon, introducing the notion of navigability of a graph. Chapter 7 focuses on another phenomenon observed in many real-world networks, namely the *power-law* distribution of the degree sequence (or number of neighbours) of the graph. The most salient feature of a sequence with a power-law distribution is that it typically contains samples with very high values. In contrast, classical network models such as the Erdős–Rényi graph have degree sequences highly concentrated around their mean. Chapter 7 describes processes for generating such power laws together with their analysis. Chapter 8 covers recent results on the threshold behaviour of classical models of epidemics on general networks, identifying thresholds with graph properties of the underlying network topology. Finally, Chapter 9 approaches the algorithmic optimisation problem of maximising the spread of an epidemic on a general network by targeting nodes that are likely to yield a large cascade of infections.

Acknowledgements

We first would like to thank Frank Kelly for encouraging us to develop our initial lecture notes into this book. We would also like to thank Diana Gillooly of Cambridge University Press for her comments and advice in improving the manuscript.

PART I

SHAPELESS NETWORKS

1

Galton–Watson branching processes

1.1 Introduction

The branching process model was introduced by Sir Francis Galton in 1873
to represent the genealogical descendance of individuals. More generally it
provides a versatile model for the growth of a population of reproducing individuals in the absence of external limiting factors. It is an adequate starting
point when studying epidemics since, as we shall see in Chapter 2, it describes
accurately the early stages of an epidemic outbreak. In addition, our treatment
of so-called *dual* branching processes paves the way for the analysis of the *supercritical* phase in Chapter 2. Finally, the present chapter gives an opportunity
to introduce *large deviations* inequalities (and notably the celebrated Chernoff
bound), which is instrumental throughout the book.

A Galton–Watson branching process can be represented by a tree in which
each node represents an individual, and is linked to its parent as well as its
children. The "root" of the tree corresponds to the "ancestor" of the whole
population. An example of such a tree is depicted in Figure 1.1.

In the following we consider three distinct ways of exploring the so-called
Galton–Watson tree, each well suited to establishing specific properties.

In the *depth-first* view, we start by exploring one child in the first generation,
then explore using the same method recursively the subtree of its descendants,
before we move to the next child of the first generation. This view is used to
establish fixed-point equations satisfied by quantities of interest, such as the
extinction probability or the probability distribution of the total population.

The *breadth-first* view stems from the standard breadth-first search of trees
and graphs. It consists of exploring first the children of the root, then the children of these children, and so on. In other words, the population is explored
generation by generation. This method of exploration allows us to characterise exactly the extinction probability. In particular we will show that the

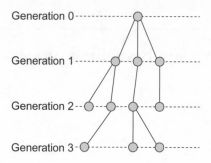

Figure 1.1 Galton–Watson branching process

population can either grow indefinitely (the supercritical case) or go extinct (the subcritical case) depending on whether the mean number of children per individual is above or below 1. This kind of behaviour, namely a qualitative change in global behaviour driven by a tiny change in a system parameter, is known as a phase transition and is widely studied in statistical physics. The emergence of unlimited population growth as the mean number of children goes above 1 is arguably the simplest example of phase transition. Several other examples will be discussed and analysed throughout the book.

Finally, the *one-by-one* view consists of exploring individual nodes' direct children starting from the ancestor. It is used to introduce the notion of dual branching processes. This duality property corresponds to a one-to-one mapping between supercritical and subcritical processes. We will also use one-by-one exploration in our study of Erdős–Rényi graphs in Chapter 2. The one-by-one view yields a description of the total population of branching processes in terms of random walks, which in turn provides simple characterisations of the total population size.

Let us now define formally the object of interest in this chapter. The Galton–Watson branching process is characterised by the probability distribution of the number of children (also called offspring) of each individual. It is a distribution on $\mathbb{N}$, denoted $\{p_k\}_{k\in\mathbb{N}}$. Starting from one individual (ancestor) at generation 0 and denoting by X_n the number of individuals at generation n, one then has

$$X_{n+1} = \sum_{i=1}^{X_n} \xi_{n,i} \, , \qquad (1.1)$$

where $\xi_{n,i}$ is the number of children of the ith individual of the nth generation.

By assumption, the $\{\xi_{n,i}\}_{i,n\in\mathbb{N}}$ are independent and identically distributed (i.i.d.), distributed according to $\{p_k\}_{k\in\mathbb{N}}$; that is, for all $k \geq 0$, $\mathbf{P}(\xi = k) = p_k$.

Now draw the tree, as in Figure 1.1, where there is one edge from each individual to each of its children. This is the so-called Galton–Watson tree. In graph-theoretic terms it is an oriented tree spanning the descendants of the ancestor and rooted at the ancestor. We shall denote this tree by $\mathcal{T}$.

1.2 Depth-first exploration

Considering depth-first exploration of the tree $\mathcal{T}$, we observe that for any child of the root, the subtree rooted at this child has the same statistical properties as $\mathcal{T}$. Thus conditional on X_1 (the number of children of the ancestor), $\mathcal{T}$ is obtained by connecting the root to the individual roots of X_1 rooted trees, $\mathcal{T}_1, \ldots, \mathcal{T}_{X_1}$, that are mutually independent, and distributed as $\mathcal{T}$.

Denote by p_{ext} the extinction probability, i.e. the probability that after some finite n, $X_n = 0$. Denote by $|\mathcal{T}|$ the number of nodes of the tree $\mathcal{T}$. We thus have

$$p_{\text{ext}} = \mathbf{P}(|\mathcal{T}| < \infty)$$

$$= \sum_{k=0}^{\infty} p_k\, \mathbf{P}(|\mathcal{T}_1| < \infty, \ldots, |\mathcal{T}_k| < \infty)$$

$$= \sum_{k=0}^{\infty} p_k p_{\text{ext}}^k .$$

Thus, denoting by

$$\phi_\xi(s) := \sum_{k\in\mathbb{N}} p_k s^k, \quad s \in \mathbb{R}$$

the generating function of the offspring distribution, the extinction probability p_{ext} is a solution of the equation

$$x = \phi_\xi(x) . \tag{1.2}$$

A similar argument yields the following result.

Theorem 1.1 (Total population) *Consider X, the total population of the branching process, given by $X = \sum_{k=0}^{\infty} X_k$. Let ϕ_X denote its generating function. Then*

$$\phi_X(s) = s\phi_\xi(\phi_X(s)) . \tag{1.3}$$

Proof Conditional on the event $X_1 = k$, i.e. that there are k individuals in the first generation, let X_j, $j = 1, \ldots, k$ denote the total number of descendents of the jth child in the first generation (also counting the jth child itself). The variables $(X_j)_{j=1,\ldots,k}$ are i.i.d. with law equal to that of X. Moreover,

$$X = 1 + \sum_{j=1}^{k} X_j \, .$$

Hence

$$\phi_X(s) := \mathbf{E}(s^X)$$
$$= \sum_{k \geq 0} p_k \, \mathbf{E}(s^X \mid X_1 = k)$$
$$= \sum_{k \geq 0} p_k \, \mathbf{E}(s^{1 + \sum_{j=1}^{k} X_j} \mid X_1 = k)$$
$$= \sum_{k \geq 0} p_k s \, \mathbf{E}(s^X)^k = s \phi_\xi(\phi_X(s)).$$

$\square$

In Section 1.4 we provide a characterisation of the total population X in terms of the sequence of numbers of children, $\{\xi_{n,i}\}_{i,n \in \mathbb{N}}$, and use it to obtain explicit bounds on the probability that the total population exceeds any particular size.

1.3 Breadth-first exploration

The breadth-first view consists of drawing the tree generation after generation. This viewpoint, which is reflected by the defining equation (1.1), allows us to characterise exactly the extinction probability p_{ext} previously introduced. We will study the existence of solutions of the equation $s = \phi_\xi(s)$ on $[0, 1]$ and characterise them in terms of the offspring distribution $\{p_k\}_{k \geq 0}$.

Theorem 1.2 (Survival vs. extinction) *The extinction probability p_{ext} is the smallest solution of equation (1.2) in $[0, 1]$. Denoting by $\mu := \mathbf{E}(\xi)$ the average number of children per individual, one further has the following regimes:*

  (i) *Subcritical regime: If $\mu < 1$, then $p_{\text{ext}} = 1$.*
  (ii) *Critical regime: If $\mu = 1$ and $p_1 < 1$, then $p_{\text{ext}} = 1$.*
  (iii) *Supercritical regime: If $\mu > 1$, then $p_{\text{ext}} < 1$.*

Proof Let $p_{\text{ext}}^{(n)} = \mathbf{P}(X_n = 0)$ be the probability that extinction has occurred at or before the nth generation. The sequence of events $(\{X_n = 0\})_{n \geq 0}$ is increasing, i.e. $\{X_n = 0\} \subseteq \{X_{n+1} = 0\}$, and converges as n goes to infinity to the extinction event. Thus the probability $p_{\text{ext}}^{(n)} := \mathbf{P}(X_n = 0)$ must converge to p_{ext} as $n \to \infty$. Let $\phi_n(s) := \mathbf{E}(s^{X_n})$. Then $\mathbf{P}(X_n = 0) = \phi_n(0)$. Using the i.i.d. property of the sequence of offspring of distinct individuals, we have

$$\phi_n(s) = \mathbf{E}(s^{X_n}) = \sum_{k=0}^{\infty} \mathbf{E}(s^{X_n} \mid X_1 = k) p_k$$

$$= \sum_{k=0}^{\infty} \left(\mathbf{E}(s^{X_{n-1}}) \right)^k p_k \, .$$

Taking $s = 0$ yields $p_{\text{ext}}^{(n)} = \phi_\xi(p_{\text{ext}}^{(n-1)})$.

Let us prove that p_{ext} is the smallest solution of equation (1.2) in $[0, 1]$. Let $\psi \in [0, 1]$ be a solution of equation (1.2). First note that $p_{\text{ext}}^{(0)} = 0 \leq \psi$. Then, by induction and using the monotonicity of ϕ_ξ on $[0, 1]$ (which holds in view of the expression $\phi_\xi'(s) = \sum_{k \geq 1} k p_k s^{k-1}$), we have that $p_{\text{ext}}^{(n)} \leq \psi$ for $n \geq 0$ and, by taking the limit when n goes to infinity, $p_{\text{ext}} \leq \psi$.

Let us now use this characterisation to establish properties of p_{ext}. Note first that the function ϕ_ξ is non-decreasing and convex ($\phi_\xi''(s) = \sum_{k \geq 2} k(k-1)s^{k-2} p_k$ is non-negative on $[0, 1]$), and such that its derivative $\phi_\xi'(1)$ equals the average number of children, μ. It is moreover strictly convex whenever $p_0 + p_1 < 1$.

In the case where $p_0 = 0$, necessarily $p_{\text{ext}} = 0$ is the smallest solution. This can also be seen directly: each individual has at least one child, so the process survives forever.

Assume now that $p_0 > 0$. Since $\{p_k\}_{k \geq 0}$ is a probability distribution, necessarily $p_1 < 1$.

Consider then the following cases.

(i) $\mu < 1$: In this case $\phi_\xi'(1) = \mu < 1$ so that, for small enough $\epsilon > 0$, $\phi_\xi(1 - \epsilon) \sim 1 - \mu\epsilon > 1 - \epsilon$. Thus, by convexity of ϕ_ξ, the only solution of equation (1.2) is $x = 1$ so that $p_{\text{ext}} = 1$.

(ii) $\mu = 1$: Here the previous assumption that $p_0 > 0$ is equivalent to $p_1 < 1$. In this situation, $p_0 + p_1 < 1$ so that ϕ_ξ is strictly convex. It is therefore strictly above its tangent at $x = 1$, whose equation is $y = 1 + \mu(x - 1)$ or equivalently $y = x$. Thus the only solution to equation (1.2) is again $x = 1$.

(iii) $\mu > 1$: In this case, for small enough $\epsilon > 0$, $\phi_\xi(1 - \epsilon) \sim 1 - \mu\epsilon < 1 - \epsilon$. Thus by continuity of the function $x \to \phi_\xi(x) - x$, which takes a positive value p_0 at $x = 0$ and a negative value at $x = 1 - \epsilon$, there must exist a solution to equation (1.2) in $[0, 1 - \epsilon]$. Therefore its smallest solution p_{ext} must be strictly less than 1.

$\square$

For example, consider a Galton–Watson branching process with Poisson offspring distribution with parameter $\lambda > 1$, i.e. $p_k = e^{-\lambda}\lambda^k/k!$, $k \geq 0$. The corresponding extinction probability is then the smallest solution in $[0, 1]$ of $x = e^{\lambda(x-1)}$.

1.4 One-by-one exploration

Now consider the following construction of the Galton–Watson tree. Throughout the exploration one keeps track of a number of so-called *active* nodes, meaning that they have been unveiled by our exploration but their children have not yet been unveiled. Starting with the ancestor as the only active node, each step of the exploration consists of the following. One picks in an arbitrary fashion some active node, unveils its children (who thus become active) and deactivates the originally selected active node.

Denoting by A_n the number of active nodes at step n, and by ξ_n the number of children of the node chosen at step n, one has the recursion

$$\begin{aligned} A_0 &= 1, \\ A_n &= A_{n-1} - 1 + \xi_n, \quad n \geq 0. \end{aligned} \tag{1.4}$$

The ξ_n in this expression are i.i.d., distributed according to the offspring distribution $\{p_k\}_{k\geq 0}$. Thus the $\{A_n\}_{n\geq 0}$ constitute a random walk with i.i.d. increments $\xi_n - 1$.

This exploration of the tree stops when there are no longer any active nodes, i.e. at step $\mathcal{Y}$, where

$$\mathcal{Y} = \inf\{n > 0 : A_n = 0\}.$$

In other words, it stops when the whole population has been explored; therefore, $\mathcal{Y}$ coincides with the total population $\mathcal{X}$ introduced in Theorem 1.1. It is easily seen by induction that $A_n = 1 + \sum_{i=1}^{n} \xi_i - n$. Using the fact that $A_{\mathcal{X}} = 0$, it follows that

$$\mathcal{X} = 1 + \sum_{i=1}^{\mathcal{X}} \xi_i.$$

Note that the right-hand side counts the ancestor plus the number of children of each node in the Galton–Watson tree. Therefore, $\mathcal{X}$ equals the total number of individuals in the Galton–Watson tree.

We now formalise the above description by defining the so-called *history* of a branching process.

Definition 1.3 (History of a branching process)　The *history* of a branching process is given by the sequence $H = \{\xi_0, \xi_1, \ldots, \xi_X\}$ of numbers of children discovered in the one-by-one exploration described above. It thus satisfies the constraints

$$A_n > 0, \quad n = 0, \ldots, X - 1,$$
$$A_X = 0,$$

where the A_n are given by (1.4).

Note that the history H admits the following distribution. For any finite sequence $x_1, \ldots, x_T$ that constitutes a history, one has

$$\mathbf{P}(H = (x_1, \ldots, x_k)) = \prod_{i=1}^{k} p_{x_i}. \tag{1.5}$$

We shall now relate the distribution of a supercritical branching process conditioned on extinction to an (unconditioned) dual subcritical branching process.

Fix a reference (critical) offspring distribution $\{q_k\}_{k \geq 0}$ such that $q_0 > 0$ and $\sum_{k \geq 0} k q_k = 1$. Let $\lambda > 0$ be a parameter and define the corresponding *exponentially tilted* distribution $\{p_k(\lambda)\}_{k \geq 0}$ by

$$p_k(\lambda) = q_k \frac{\lambda^k}{\phi(\lambda)} ,$$

where $\phi(\lambda) := \sum_{k \geq 0} q_k \lambda^k$. It is easy to see that this is a probability distribution and that $\lambda > 1$ corresponds to the offspring distribution of a supercritical branching process, whereas $\lambda < 1$ corresponds to the offspring distribution of a subcritical branching process.

Example 1.4　With $q_k = e^{-1}/k!$ the unit-mean Poisson distribution, one has $\phi(\lambda) = e^{-1+\lambda}$, and thus the tilted distribution $p_k(\lambda)$ is the Poisson distribution with parameter λ.

We now define a duality relation between the average number of children of two distinct branching processes.

Definition 1.5 (Dual or conjugate parameter)　Given the reference distribution $\{q_k\}_{k \geq 0}$, one says that parameter μ is *dual (or conjugate)* to λ if

$$\frac{\phi(\lambda)}{\lambda} = \frac{\phi(\mu)}{\mu} .$$

We now illustrate how to derive the conjugate of a given parameter.

Proposition 1.6 *Given a parameter $\lambda > 1$, there is a unique conjugate parameter $\mu \neq \lambda$. It satisfies $\mu < 1$ and is given by*

$$\mu = \lambda p_{\text{ext}}(\lambda), \tag{1.6}$$

where $p_{\text{ext}}(\lambda)$ is the extinction probability associated with the offspring distribution $\{p_k(\lambda)\}_{k \geq 0}$.

Proof The function $f(x) := \phi(x)/x = \sum_{k \geq 0} q_k x^{k-1}$ is strictly convex on $\mathbb{R}_+$ because $q_0 > 0$. Moreover $f(1) = 1$, $f'(1) = 0$ and $f(0^+) = +\infty$. Therefore there is a unique $\mu \neq \lambda$ such that $f(\mu) = f(\lambda)$, and it is necessarily strictly less than 1.

Note now that $p_{\text{ext}}(\lambda) = \sum_{k \geq 0} p_k(\lambda)(p_{\text{ext}}(\lambda))^k$. Using the expression of $p_k(\lambda)$ in terms of q_k, it follows that

$$\frac{\phi(\lambda)}{\lambda} = \frac{\phi(\lambda p_{\text{ext}}(\lambda))}{\lambda p_{\text{ext}}(\lambda)} ,$$

i.e. that $\lambda p_{\text{ext}}(\lambda)$ is dual to λ. By Theorem 1.2, $p_{\text{ext}}(\lambda) < 1$. Thus $\lambda p_{\text{ext}}(\lambda)$ is the unique parameter dual to λ and distinct from it. $\qquad\square$

Theorem 1.7 *Let $\lambda > 1$ be fixed. The distribution of the history $\{\xi_1, \ldots, \xi_X\}$ under offspring distribution $\{p_k(\lambda)\}_{k \geq 0}$, conditioned on extinction, coincides with the distribution of the history under offspring distribution $\{p_k(\mu)\}_{k \geq 0}$, where $\mu = \lambda p_{\text{ext}}(\lambda)$ is the dual parameter of λ.*

Proof Let a finite history $\{\xi_1, \ldots, \xi_X\}$ be given. By definition, one necessarily has $\sum_{i=1}^{X} \xi_i = X - 1$. Thus the probability of this history under offspring distribution $\{p_k(\lambda)\}_{k \geq 0}$, conditioned on extinction, i.e. that the total population is finite, is

$$\mathbf{P}(H \mid \text{Extinction}) = \frac{1}{p_{\text{ext}}(\lambda)} \prod_{i=1}^{X} p_{\xi_i}(\lambda)$$

$$= \frac{1}{p_{\text{ext}}(\lambda)} \prod_{i=1}^{X} q_{\xi_i} \frac{\lambda^{\xi_i}}{\phi_1(\lambda)}$$

$$= \frac{1}{p_{\text{ext}}(\lambda)} \frac{\lambda^{X-1}}{\phi_1(\lambda)^X} \prod_{i=1}^{X} q_{\xi_i}$$

$$= \frac{\mu^{X-1}}{\phi_1(\mu)^X} \prod_{i=1}^{X} q_{\xi_i}$$

$$= \prod_{i=1}^{X} p_{\xi_i}(\mu) ,$$

where we use the duality relation between λ and μ. The last expression is precisely the probability of history H under the offspring distribution $\{p_k(\mu)\}_{k\geq0}$.

□

Since the extinction event involves all the individual numbers of children in a branching process, it is not obvious a priori that the behaviour of a supercritical process, conditioned on extinction, has a simple structure. The above duality result shows that its structure is indeed simple, namely it is that of an unconditioned subcritical branching process. Duality will also prove instrumental in the next chapter.

1.5 Chernoff bounds and total population size

The next application of the one-by-one representation of a branching process is to obtain bounds on the total population in the subcritical case $\mathbf{E}(\xi) < 1$. The main tool is the Chernoff bound.

Lemma 1.8 (Chernoff bound)   *Given i.i.d. random variables $X_1,\ldots,X_n$, for any $a \in \mathbb{R}$, one has*

$$\mathbf{P}\left(\sum_{i=1}^{n} X_i \geq na\right) \leq e^{-nh(a)},$$

where

$$h(a) = \sup_{\theta\geq0} \left[\theta a - \log \mathbf{E}(e^{\theta X_1})\right].$$

The function $h(a)$ is known as the rate function of X_1. It gives the speed of the exponential decrease of the probability $\mathbf{P}(\sum_{i=1}^{n} X_i \geq na)$ as n tends to infinity.

Proof   For all $\theta \geq 0$, by Chebyshev's inequality, one has

$$\mathbf{P}\left(\sum_{i=1}^{n} X_i \geq na\right) = \mathbf{P}\left(\exp\left(\theta \sum_{i=1}^{n} X_i\right) \geq \exp(n\theta a)\right)$$

$$\leq \mathbf{E}\left[\exp\left(\theta \sum_{i=1}^{n} X_i\right)\right] e^{-n\theta a}$$

$$\leq \exp\left(-n\left[\theta a - \log \mathbf{E}(e^{\theta X_1})\right]\right).$$

The result follows by optimising this bound over $\theta \geq 0$.

□

The Chernoff bound is useful when there exists some $b > 0$ such that $\mathbf{E}[\exp(bX_1)] < +\infty$ and $a > \mathbf{E}(X_1)$. Under the first condition, the function

$\theta \to \theta a - \log \mathbf{E}[\exp(\theta X_1)]$ is finite and differentiable in the interval $[0, b)$. Its derivative at $\theta = 0^+$ equals $a - \mathbf{E}(X_1)$, which is positive under the second condition. Thus under the two conditions, the exponent $h(a)$ is strictly positive.

A direct application of the Chernoff bound yields:

Lemma 1.9 *The total population X of the branching process satisfies*

$$\mathbf{P}(X > k) \leq \exp(-k h(1)),$$

where $h(x) = \sup_{\theta \geq 0} [\theta x - \log \mathbf{E}(\exp(\theta \xi))]$.

Proof One-by-one exploration results in the sequence of active numbers of nodes, $A_0, A_1, \ldots, A_X$, where X is the total population size and is also the first step t at which A_t equals 0. For each $t \leq X$, the number A_t reads

$$A_t = 1 + \sum_{i=1}^{t} \xi_i, \tag{1.7}$$

where $\{\xi_1, \ldots, \xi_X\}$ is the corresponding history of the process.

We can extend the sequence $\{\xi_i\}$ to any positive index i, while retaining its i.i.d. property, by padding it with additional variables ξ_i, $i > X$, themselves i.i.d. and distributed according to the offspring distribution $\{p_k\}_{k \geq 0}$. In turn, we extend the sequence $\{A_t\}$ to arbitrary indices $t \geq 0$ via the formula (1.7).

The resulting sequence $\{A_t\}_{t \geq 0}$ then becomes a standard random walk, originating at 1, with independent increments distributed according to $\{p_k\}_{k \geq 0}$. The total population X is then defined as the hitting time of 0 by this random walk.

One thus has

$$\mathbf{P}(X \geq k) = \mathbf{P}(A_1 > 0, \ldots, A_k > 0)$$
$$\leq \mathbf{P}(A_k > 0)$$
$$= \mathbf{P}\left(A_0 + \sum_{i=1}^{k} \xi_i > k\right)$$
$$= \mathbf{P}\left(\sum_{i=1}^{k} \xi_i \geq k\right).$$

The claimed bound then follows directly from the Chernoff bound. □

Example 1.10 If the offspring distribution is Poisson(λ), one has

$$h(x) = \sup_{\theta \geq 0} \left[\theta x - \log \left(\sum_{k \geq 0} e^{-\lambda} \frac{(\lambda e^\theta)^k}{k!} \right) \right]$$
$$= \sup_{\theta \geq 0} \left[\theta x - \lambda(e^\theta - 1) \right].$$

Upon differentiating the function $\theta \to \theta x - \lambda(e^\theta - 1)$, one finds that the maximum is reached at $\theta = \log(x/\lambda)$, giving

$$h(x) = \lambda h_1(x/\lambda),$$

where $h_1(u) = u \log(u) - u + 1$.

1.6 Notes

Branching processes are an important and well-studied class of random processes. A general treatment is provided in the book by Harris [40]. For a survey of the history of their invention by Sir Francis Galton, one can check http://galton.org/. The characterisation of the extinction probability is perhaps the most classical result. The duality and the one-by-one exploration covered in this chapter are less standard, and are introduced to pave the way for Chapter 2.

1.7 Problems

1. *Geometric branching process:* Consider a Galton–Watson branching process with geometric offspring distribution with parameter p, i.e.

$$\mathbf{P}(\xi = k) = p^k(1 - p).$$

   (i) Compute the probability of extinction occurring in generation n (using generating functions).
   (ii) Give a general expression for the probability of extinction.
   (iii) Derive an expression for the generating function of

$$W = \lim_{n \to \infty} X_n/(\mathbf{E}(\xi))^n,$$

   where X_n is the number of individuals in generation n.

2. *Conditioned branching process:* Consider a supercritical branching process with offspring distribution p_k and generating function ϕ.

   Prove that if we condition on non-extinction and consider individuals who have an infinite line of descent then the corresponding branching process has offspring distribution

$$\tilde{\phi}(s) = \frac{\phi((1 - p_{\text{ext}})s + p_{\text{ext}}) - p_{\text{ext}}}{1 - p_{\text{ext}}}.$$

Hint: Prove that the number of individuals in the first generation who have an infinite line of descent has distribution

$$\tilde{p}_j = \frac{1}{1 - p_{\text{ext}}} \sum_{k \geq j} p_k \binom{k}{j} (1 - p_{\text{ext}})^j p_{\text{ext}}^{k-j}.$$

3. *Multitype Poisson branching process:* Let Λ be an ℓ by ℓ matrix with non-negative entries λ_{ij}. The branching process $B_i(\Lambda)$, $1 \leq i \leq \ell$, is defined as follows: start with a single ancestor of type i in generation 0. Each particle of type i has for each j a Poisson number of children of type j, with mean λ_{ij}. The number of children of different types of a given ancestor are independent, as are the numbers of children of different individuals. Let $p_i = \mathbf{P}(B_i(\Lambda) = \infty)$.

   (i) Show that the vector $(p_1, \ldots, p_\ell)$ is the solution of

$$p_i = 1 - \exp\left(-\sum_{j=1}^{\ell} \lambda_{ij} p_j\right),$$

such that $p_i \geq 0$, and that for any other solution $(q_1, \ldots, q_\ell)$, $p_i \geq q_i$ for every i.
   (ii) Compute the expected value of the kth generation of $B_i(\Lambda)$.
   (iii) State and prove a necessary and sufficient condition on Λ for $\sum_i p_i$ to be positive.

4. *Chernoff bound:* Let $X_1, \ldots, X_n$ be independent $\{0, 1\}$ random variables such that $\mu = \mathbf{E} \sum_{i=1}^{n} X_i$. Let $X = \sum_{i=1}^{n} X_i$. Prove the following inequalities:
   (i) For any $0 < \delta \leq 1$, $\mathbf{P}(|X - \mu| \geq \delta\mu) \leq 2e^{-\mu\delta^2/3}$.
   (ii) For $R \geq 6\mu$, $\mathbf{P}(X \geq R) \leq 2^{-R}$.

5. *Chernoff bound continued:* Suppose X_i are independent random variables satisfying $X_i \leq M$, for all i, $M > 0$. Let $X = \sum_{i=1}^{n} X_i$ and $\|X\| = \sqrt{\sum_{i=1}^{n} \mathbf{E}X_i^2}$.
   (i) Prove that, for $\lambda > 0$

$$\mathbf{P}(X \geq \mathbf{E}X + \lambda) \leq \exp\left(-\frac{\lambda^2}{2(\|X\|^2 + M\lambda/3)}\right).$$

   (ii) Describe how you would prove a similar result for $|X - \mathbf{E}X|$ when $|X_i| \leq M$, for all i.

2

Reed–Frost epidemics and Erdős–Rényi random graphs

2.1 Introduction

The Reed–Frost model is a particular example of an SIR (susceptible-infective-removed) epidemic process. It is one of the earliest stochastic SIR models to be studied in depth, because of its analytical tractability. In the general SIR model, the population initially consists of healthy individuals and a small number of infected individuals. Infected individuals encounter healthy individuals in a random fashion for a given period known as the infectious period and then are removed and cease spreading the epidemic. Alternatively, in the context of rumour spreading, healthy individuals correspond to nodes that ignore the rumour whereas infected individuals are nodes that initially hold the rumour and actively pass it on to others. Removed individuals correspond to nodes that cease spreading the rumour, or stiflers.

The Reed–Frost epidemic corresponds to a discrete-time version of the SIR model where the infectious period lasts one unit of time. Another commonly used model assumes that infectious periods are independent and identically distributed (i.i.d.) according to an exponential distribution, so that the system evolves as a continuous-time Markov process. This continuous-time SIR model is amenable to the analysis presented in Chapter 5 whereby the dynamics of the Markovian epidemic process is approximated by the solution of a set of differential equations.

The basic version of the Reed–Frost model is as follows. A set of n individuals is given, indexed by $i \in \{1, \ldots, n\}$. At step 0, a single individual is infected. Once infected, an individual is infectious during the subsequent time slot, after which it is removed (either dead or immunised). While infectious, it will succeed in infecting a healthy individual with probability p, and this independently for all target individuals and infectious individuals. Thus the model's parameters are the number of individuals, or nodes, n, and the infection probability, p.

A more formal description is as follows. Let $Z_u(t) \in \{S, I, R\}$ denote the state of node u during step t. Then the process $Z(t) = \{Z_u(t)\}_{u \in \{1,\dots,n\}}$ is a homogeneous discrete-time Markov process; i.e. conditional on its state $Z(t)$ at time t, the future evolution of the process after t is independent of the states visited prior to t. Given two states z, z' in $\{S, I, R\}^n$, a transition from z to z' can take place only if for all $i = 1, \dots, n$, $z_i \in \{I, R\} \Rightarrow z_i' = R$: all nodes are removed after being infected, and remain removed afterwards; and $z_i = S \Rightarrow z_i' \in \{S, I\}$. Denoting $I(z)$ (resp. $S(z)$, $R(z)$) the number of infectious (resp. susceptible, removed) nodes in state z, provided the pair of states z, z' satisfies the above constraints, one can check that the transition probability is given by

$$\mathbf{P}(Z(t+1) = z' \mid Z(t) = z) = \binom{S(z)}{I(z')}(1-p)^{I(z)S(z')}[1 - (1-p)^{I(z)}]^{I(z')}.$$

Note that $I(z') = S(z) - S(z')$.

A closely related model is provided by the Erdős–Rényi (E-R) random graph. The E-R random graph denoted $G(n, p)$ is defined as follows. It is a graph on n nodes $\{1, \dots, n\}$, in which for each pair (u, v) of nodes, $u < v$, the edge (u, v) is present with probability p, independently of the presence of other edges. Let $\xi_{uv} = 1$ if edge (u, v) is present and $\xi_{uv} = 0$ otherwise.

The Reed–Frost epidemic can then be constructed from the $G(n, p)$ model, in the following manner. Assume node u is infected during step t. Then for any other node v, u will successfully infect v during step $t + 1$ if $\xi_{uv} = 1$ (assuming case $u < v$; if $v < u$, use the variable ξ_{vu} instead). Note that if the target node v is already infected or removed, it will already have "used" the random variable ξ_{uv}, but this is of no consequence since then node u can no longer infect v.

The corresponding state of the Reed–Frost epidemic at time t, if initiated from a single infectious node $u \in \{1, \dots, n\}$, can be described purely in terms of graph-theoretic properties of $G(n, p)$.

Let $d_G(u, v)$ denote the shortest number of hops in a path connecting u to v in the graph G, i.e. the graph distance between u and v. Define the i-neighbourhood of node u as

$$\Gamma_i(u) := \{v : d_{G(n,p)}(u, v) = i\}.$$

Then the state of the Reed–Frost epidemic started at u, at time t, is given by

$$Z_v(t) = R \text{ if } d_{G(n,p)}(u, v) < t,$$
$$Z_v(t) = I \text{ if } d_{G(n,p)}(u, v) = t, \text{ i.e. if } v \in \Gamma_t(u),$$
$$Z_v(t) = S \text{ otherwise}.$$

Let us denote by $C(u)$ the connected component of the graph to which node u belongs, i.e. the set of nodes connected to u by some path. Thus in the Reed–Frost epidemic started at node u, the set of nodes that are eventually removed is precisely the connected component $C(u)$.

The E-R random graph is a highly stylised, symmetrical model that does not capture the statistical properties of real-world networks. Nevertheless, it displays interesting behaviour that will be relevant when we analyse more involved structures in the second part of this book (Part II: Structured Networks). Examining this graph will enable us to introduce a number of important notions: the emergence of a giant component in the present chapter, connectivity and atomic infection in Chapter 3, diameter and time to atomic infection in Chapter 4 and the small-world phenomenon in Chapter 6.

We will revisit the SIR model with heterogeneous mixing, i.e. with nonuniform infection probabilities, in the context of general graphs in Chapter 8.

In this chapter we study the size of connected components in an E-R graph. In particular we shall determine under which conditions *a giant component*, i.e. a component containing a non-negligible fraction of the whole population, appears. We will identify three different phases, corresponding to the size of the largest connected component being (i) logarithmic in n (the subcritical phase, with no giant component), (ii) linear in n (the subcritical phase, with the existence of a giant component) and (iii) of order $n^{2/3}$ (the critical phase), depending on the value of p as a function of n. The proof, in all three cases, will be based on the fact that, for large n, the E-R graph (and consequently the Reed–Frost epidemic) can be described in terms of a Galton–Watson branching process.

2.2 Emergence of the giant component

We now study the size of the largest component of the graph $G(n, p)$ as $n \to \infty$, assuming the parameter p depends on n in such a way that $np \equiv \lambda > 0$ as $n \to \infty$. Denote by C_1 the largest connected component of $G(n, p)$ (the size being measured in number of constituent nodes), by C_2 the second largest component, etc. For any subset C of $\{1, \ldots, n\}$, we will denote by $|C|$ the number of elements in C.

Theorem 2.1 *Depending on the value of λ, the following regimes occur.*

(i) $\lambda < 1$: Subcritical regime. For some constant a depending on λ, the

following holds:

$$\lim_{n\to\infty} \mathbf{P}\left(|C_1| \le a\log(n)\right) = 1. \tag{2.1}$$

(ii) $\lambda > 1$: *Supercritical regime. Denote by* $p_{\text{ext}}(\lambda)$ *the extinction probability of a Galton–Watson branching process with Poisson(λ) offspring distribution, i.e. the unique root in $(0, 1)$ of the equation* $x = \exp(-\lambda(1 - x))$. *Then for some constant* $a' > 0$ *depending on* λ, *and all* $\delta > 0$, *one has the following:*

$$\lim_{n\to\infty} \mathbf{P}\left(\left|\frac{|C_1|}{n} - (1 - p_{\text{ext}}(\lambda))\right| \le \delta \text{ and } |C_2| \le a'\log(n)\right) = 1. \tag{2.2}$$

(iii) $\lambda = 1$: *Critical regime. There is a constant* $\kappa > 0$ *such that, for all* $a > 0$, *one has the following:*

$$\mathbf{P}(|C_1| \ge an^{2/3}) \le \frac{\kappa}{a^2}. \tag{2.3}$$

This theorem states that in the subcritical regime ($\lambda < 1$), all connected components are of logarithmic size; in the supercritical regime ($\lambda > 1$) a "giant" component appears, whose size scaled by n converges in probability as $n \to \infty$ to $1 - p_{\text{ext}}(\lambda)$, while other components remain of logarithmic size. In the critical regime ($\lambda = 1$) we shall only establish upper bounds on the size of the largest component, of order $n^{2/3}$. Lower bounds of matching order could be established; references are provided at the end of the chapter.

In terms of the outcome of the Reed–Frost epidemic, the subcritical case (i) results in a *small outbreak*, i.e. a negligible proportion of the population is eventually infected, whereas in the supercritical case (ii) a *large outbreak* occurs, i.e. a sizeable proportion of the population, given by the constant $1 - p_{\text{ext}}(\lambda)$, is ultimately infected.

Before we start proving these results, we first give a high-level view of the proof strategy. We will analyse the (probability distribution of the) size of an arbitrary connected component. This will be performed by using an analogue of the one-by-one exploration previously introduced in the context of Galton–Watson processes. We will show that this exploration is accurately approximated by that of a Galton–Watson process with offspring distribution that is binomial with parameters $n - 1$ and p. Such a Galton–Watson process behaves radically differently according to whether the average number of offspring $(n - 1)p$ is above or below 1. This dichotomy will be in correspondence with the different regimes identified in the theorem.

2.3 The subcritical regime

For an arbitrary node $v \in \{1, \ldots, n\}$, construct the connected component containing v, denoted $C(v)$, in the following manner, similar to the one-by-one exploration of Galton–Watson branching processes.

We maintain at any given step $k \geq 0$ two disjoint subsets of nodes from $C(v)$, namely the set $\mathcal{A}_k$ of active nodes and the set $\mathcal{B}_k$ of inactive nodes, starting with $\mathcal{A}_0 = \{v\}$ and $\mathcal{B}_0 = \emptyset$. These sets are updated as follows. At step k, one picks an arbitrary node from $\mathcal{A}_{k-1}$, say v_{k-1}. This node is then deactivated, and all its graph neighbours within $\{1, \ldots, n\} \setminus \{\mathcal{A}_{k-1} \cup \mathcal{B}_{k-1}\}$ are turned into active nodes. Denoting by $\mathcal{D}_k$ this set of newly activated neighbours, one has the following updates:

$$\mathcal{A}_k = \mathcal{A}_{k-1} \cup \mathcal{D}_k \setminus \{v_{k-1}\},$$
$$\mathcal{B}_k = \mathcal{B}_{k-1} \cup \{v_{k-1}\}.$$

Denote by A_k, B_k and ξ_k the sizes of $\mathcal{A}_k$, $\mathcal{B}_k$ and $\mathcal{D}_k$ respectively. One then has the recursion

$$A_0 = 1,$$
$$A_k = A_{k-1} - 1 + \xi_k, \ k > 0.$$

Note that, conditional on $\xi_1, \ldots, \xi_{k-1}$, the random variable ξ_k is binomially distributed, with parameters $n - k - 1 - A_{k-1}$ and p. The procedure stops when $\mathcal{A}_k$ first becomes empty. It is not hard to see that it stops precisely when all nodes in the component $C(v)$ have been found and deactivated. Let

$$X := \inf\{k > 0 : A_k = 0\}$$

be the step at which the procedure stops. Thus, as in the exploration of the Galton–Watson tree, the size of $C(v)$ satisfies

$$|C(v)| = |B_X| = X.$$

The following lemmas will be used in the proof of Theorem 2.1.

Lemma 2.2 *For $k \geq 0$, the random variable $A_k + k - 1$ admits a binomial distribution with parameters $n - 1$ and $1 - (1 - p)^k$.*

Proof Let X_k be the number of nodes that have not been identified as belonging to $C(v)$ after k steps of the exploration outlined above. It is easy to see that $X_k = n - k - A_k$. We now argue that X_k admits a binomial distribution with parameters $n - 1$ and $(1 - p)^k$. This will readily imply the lemma, since $A_k + k - 1 = n - 1 - X_k$, and for any binomial random variable X with parameters m, q, the random variable $m - X$ is binomial with parameters m and $1 - q$.

To proceed, consider the following specific construction of the consecutive sets $\mathcal{A}_i$, $\mathcal{B}_i$. Let i.i.d. Bernoulli random variables $\{Z_{i,w}\}_{i>0,w=1,\dots,n}$ be given, all with parameter p. A specific node $w \neq v$ will belong to the set $\mathcal{D}_i$ if and only if $Z_{i,w}$ equals 1 and it has not been incorporated in any of $D_1, \dots, D_{i-1}$. It can be checked that this produces a sequence of sets with the desired distribution.

Each node $w \neq v$ fails to be incorporated by step k if and only if $Z_{1,w} = \cdots = Z_{k,w} = 0$, which happens with probability $(1 - p)^k$, and this independently for all such w. Thus X_k is the sum of $n - 1$ independent $\{0, 1\}$-valued random variables, each equal to 1 with probability $(1 - p)^k$. It thus has the claimed binomial distribution.   □

Lemma 2.3   *For any $\theta > 0$,*

$$\mathbf{P}(|C(v)| > k) \leq \exp\left(-k(\theta - \lambda(1 - e^\theta))\right).$$

Proof   For fixed $\theta > 0$, applying Lemma 2.2 we have

$$\mathbf{P}(|C(v)| > k) \leq \mathbf{P}(A_k > 0) \leq \mathbf{P}(\text{Bin}(n - 1, 1 - (1 - p)^k) \geq k).$$

Since $1 - (1 - p)^k \leq kp$ and $n - 1 < n$, it is immediate to check that

$$\mathbf{P}(\text{Bin}(n - 1, 1 - (1 - p)^k) \geq k) \leq \mathbf{P}(\text{Bin}(n, kp) \geq k).$$

Hence, applying the Chernoff bounding technique, we obtain, for $\theta \geq 0$,

$$\mathbf{P}(|C(v)| > k) \leq \mathbf{P}(\text{Bin}(n, kp) \geq k) \leq \mathbf{E}\left(e^{\theta \text{Bin}(n,kp)}\right) e^{-\theta k}$$
$$= (1 - p + pe^\theta)^{nk} e^{-\theta k}$$
$$\leq \exp\left(-npk(1 - e^\theta)\right) e^{-\theta k}$$
$$= \exp\left(-k(\theta + \lambda(1 - e^\theta))\right),$$

where we use the inequality $1 + x \leq \exp(x)$, $x \geq 0$, in the penultimate step.   □

Proof of Theorem 2.1 (i)   In Lemma 2.3, for $\lambda < 1$ and θ small enough, the exponent $\theta + \lambda(1 - e^\theta)$ is positive, which ensures that there is a positive constant β such that $\mathbf{P}(|C(v)| > k) \leq e^{-\beta k}$. In fact recalling the discussion of Chernoff bounds in the previous chapter, upon optimising over θ, one can take $\beta = h(1)$, where $h(a) := a \log(a/\lambda) - a + \lambda$. Thus, for $\delta > 0$,

$$\mathbf{P}(|C_1| > \beta^{-1}(1 + \delta) \log(n)) = \mathbf{P}(\max_{i=1,\dots,n} |C(i)| > \beta^{-1}(1 + \delta) \log(n))$$
$$\leq \sum_{i=1}^n \mathbf{P}(|C(i)| > \beta^{-1}(1 + \delta) \log(n))$$
$$= n \mathbf{P}(|C(v)| > \beta^{-1}(1 + \delta) \log(n))$$
$$\leq n^{-\delta}$$

by the previous inequality. The last term tends to 0 as n goes to infinity. Therefore the probability that there is a connected component of size larger than $\beta^{-1}(1 + \delta) \log(n)$ tends to 0.

2.4 The supercritical regime

We shall need the following version of the Chernoff bound.

Lemma 2.4 *Let X be a sum of independent, not necessarily identically distributed, $\{0, 1\}$-valued random variables. Let $\bar{X} = \mathbf{E}(X)$. Then for all $\epsilon > 0$,*

$$\mathbf{P}(X - \bar{X} \geq \epsilon \bar{X}) \leq e^{-\bar{X}h(\epsilon)}, \quad \mathbf{P}(X - \bar{X} \leq -\epsilon \bar{X}) \leq e^{-\bar{X}h(-\epsilon)}, \quad (2.4)$$

where $h(x) := (1 + x) \log(1 + x) - x$.

Proof We will only prove the first inequality, as the second inequality is proved in the same way. Fix $\theta > 0$, and let $(X_i)_{i=1,\dots,n}$ be independent Bernoulli random variables such that $\mathbf{P}(X_i = 1) = 1 - \mathbf{P}(X_i = 0) = p_i$, $X = \sum_{i=1}^n X_i$ and $\bar{X} = \sum_{i=1}^n p_i$. One then has, for $\theta \geq 0$,

$$\mathbf{P}(X - \bar{X} \geq \epsilon \bar{X}) \leq \mathbf{E}(e^{\theta(X - \bar{X})}) e^{-\theta \epsilon \bar{X}}$$

$$= e^{-\theta \epsilon \bar{X}} \prod_{i=1}^n \mathbf{E}(e^{\theta(X_i - p_i)})$$

$$= e^{-\theta(1+\epsilon)\bar{X}} \prod_{i=1}^n \mathbf{E}(e^{\theta X_i})$$

$$= e^{-\theta(1+\epsilon)\bar{X}} \prod_{i=1}^n (1 + p_i(e^\theta - 1))$$

$$\leq e^{-\theta(1+\epsilon)\bar{X}} \prod_{i=1}^n e^{p_i(e^\theta - 1)}$$

$$= \exp\left(-\bar{X}(1 - e^\theta + \theta(1 + \epsilon))\right),$$

where we use the classical inequality $1 + x \leq e^x$, $x \geq 0$. To conclude we optimise over θ. $\square$

We shall also need the following ingredients.

Lemma 2.5 *Let $\lambda = np > 1$ be given. Then for all $\epsilon > 0$, there is an integer $k_0 > 0$ such that, for n large enough,*

$$p_{\text{ext}}(\lambda) - \epsilon \leq \mathbf{P}(|C(v)| < k_0) \leq p_{\text{ext}}(\lambda) + \epsilon .$$

Proof Recall the previous construction of a connected component $C(v)$, and the fact that the conditional distribution of ξ_k given $\xi_1, \ldots, \xi_{k-1}$ is binomial with parameters $(n - 1 - \xi_1 - \cdots - \xi_{k-1}, p)$.

For any fixed k, the vector $(\xi_1, \ldots, \xi_k)$ converges in distribution to a vector of independent Poisson random variables with common parameter λ, corresponding to the history of a Galton–Watson branching process with Poisson(λ) offspring distribution. Indeed, this follows from the evaluation

$$\mathbf{P}(\xi_1 = x_1, \ldots, \xi_k = x_k) = \prod_{i=1}^{k} \binom{n - 1 - \sum_{j=1}^{i-1} x_j}{x_i} p^{x_i}(1 - p)^{n-1-\sum_{j=1}^{i-1} x_j}$$

$$= (1 + o(1)) \prod_{i=1}^{k} e^{-\lambda} \frac{\lambda^{x_i}}{x_i!},$$

where the final equality is for n large. Convergence holds for all $(x_1, \ldots, x_k) \in \mathbb{N}^k$, and hence the asserted convergence in distribution $(\xi_1, \ldots, \xi_k)$ holds. This ensures the following, for all fixed $k_0 > 0$:

$$\mathbf{P}(|C(v)| \le k_0) = \mathbf{P}(\text{for some } k \le k_0, \xi_1 + \cdots + \xi_k \le k - 1)$$
$$= (1 + o(1))\mathbf{P}((\text{population size of G.W. process}$$
$$\text{with Poisson}(\lambda) \text{ offspring}) \le k_0),$$

as $n \to \infty$. Since the probability in the last line converges to $p_{\text{ext}}(\lambda)$ as k_0 increases to infinity, the result follows. $\square$

Lemma 2.6 *Let $\lambda = np > 1$ be given. Then for all $\epsilon, \delta > 0$, there is an integer $k_0 > 0$ such that, for n large enough,*

$$\mathbf{P}\Big(|C(v)| > k_0, \big||C(v)| - (1 - p_{\text{ext}}(\lambda))n\big| > \delta n\Big) \le \epsilon.$$

Proof Lemma 2.2 ensures that

$$\mathbf{P}(|C(v)| = k) \le \mathbf{P}(A_k = 0) = \mathbf{P}(X_k = k - 1), \tag{2.5}$$

where X_k has distribution $\text{Bin}(n - 1, 1 - (1 - p)^k)$.

To apply Lemma 2.4, we first need to analyse the ratio of the mean of X_k, i.e. $(n - 1)[1 - (1 - p)^k]$, to the value $k - 1$ which reads, for large n,

$$\frac{(n - 1)[1 - (1 - p)^k]}{k - 1} = (1 + o(1))\frac{n}{k}(1 - e^{-kp}) = (1 + o(1))g(k/n),$$

where $g(x) := x^{-1}[1 - e^{-\lambda x}]$. By differentiating it is easy to see that the function g is decreasing from $g(0) = \lambda > 1$ to $g(1) = 1 - e^{-\lambda}$. This readily implies the existence of a unique positive constant $x^* \in (0, 1)$ such that $g(x^*) = 1$. Since $p_{\text{ext}}(\lambda)$ is the unique solution in $(0, 1)$ of $x = e^{-\lambda(1-x)}$, then $x^* = 1 - p_{\text{ext}}(\lambda)$. Hence, for $\delta > 0$, there is a $\kappa \in (0, 1)$ such that:

- For $k \leq (1 - p_{\text{ext}}(\lambda) - \delta)n$, we have

$$\frac{k}{(n-1)[1-(1-p)^k]} < 1 - \kappa. \tag{2.6}$$

Therefore, by (2.5) and Lemma 2.4,

$$\begin{aligned}
\mathbf{P}(|C(v)| = k) &\leq \mathbf{P}(X_k \leq k) \\
&\leq \mathbf{P}(X_k - \mathbf{E}(X_k) \leq -\kappa \mathbf{E}(X_k)) \\
&\leq \exp(-\mathbf{E}(X_k)h(-\kappa)) \\
&< e^{-kh(-\kappa)},
\end{aligned}$$

where we use the fact that $\mathbf{E}(X_k) = (n-1)[1-(1-p)^k] > k$ to obtain the last inequality.

- For $k \geq (1 - p_{\text{ext}}(\lambda) + \delta)n$, we have

$$1 + \kappa < \frac{k-1}{(n-1)[1-(1-p)^k]}. \tag{2.7}$$

Therefore, by (2.5) and Lemma 2.4,

$$\begin{aligned}
\mathbf{P}(|C(v)| = k) &\leq \mathbf{P}(X_k \geq k - 1) \\
&\leq \mathbf{P}(X_k - \mathbf{E}(X_k) \geq \kappa \mathbf{E}(X_k)) \\
&\leq \exp(-\mathbf{E}(X_k)h(\kappa)) \\
&< e^{-k\theta h(\kappa)},
\end{aligned}$$

where

$$\theta = \inf_{(1-p_{ext}(\lambda)+\delta)n \leq k \leq n} \frac{\mathbf{E}(X_k)}{k},$$

the upper bound on k comes from the fact that $|C(v)|$ contains n nodes at most. Moreover, note that

$$\begin{aligned}
\mathbf{E}(X_k) &= (n-1)[1-(1-p)^k] \\
&\geq (n-1)(1-e^{-pk}) \\
&\geq (k-1)(1-e^{-\lambda(1-p_{\text{ext}}(\lambda))}),
\end{aligned}$$

where we use the fact that $\lambda = np$ together with the inequalities $1 - p_{\text{ext}}(\lambda) \leq k/n \leq 1$ in the last step. Hence, for large n, θ is bounded away from zero, being at least $1 - e^{-\lambda(1-p_{\text{ext}}(\lambda))}$, and

$$\mathbf{P}(|C(v)| = k) \leq \exp\left(-k(1 - e^{-\lambda(1-p_{\text{ext}}(\lambda))})h(\kappa)\right).$$

To sum up, we showed that, for large n,

$$\mathbf{P}(|C(v)| = k) \leq e^{-k\kappa'}, \tag{2.8}$$

where

$$\kappa' = \min\left((1 - e^{-\lambda(1-p_{\text{ext}}(\lambda))})h(\kappa), h(-\kappa)\right) > 0.$$

Now write

$$\mathbf{P}\left(|C(v)| > k_0, \left||C(v)| - (1 - p_{\text{ext}}(\lambda))n\right| > n\delta\right) \leq \sum_{k=k_0}^{(1-p_{\text{ext}}(\lambda)-\delta)n} \mathbf{P}(|C(v)| = k)$$

$$+ \sum_{k=(1-p_{\text{ext}}(\lambda)+\delta)n}^{n} \mathbf{P}(|C(v)| = k).$$

Using the bound (2.8), we have that

$$\mathbf{P}\left(|C(v)| > k_0, \left||C(v)| - (1 - p_{\text{ext}}(\lambda))n\right| > \delta n\right) \leq \sum_{k \geq k_0} e^{-\kappa' k} = \frac{e^{-\kappa' k_0}}{1 - e^{-\kappa'}},$$

for the above choice of the constant $\kappa' > 0$. Hence, for sufficiently large k_0, this quantity can be made arbitrarily small, and the lemma follows. □

Proof of Theorem 2.1 (ii) To conclude the proof of Theorem 2.1 (ii) we analyse the following algorithm for identifying the giant component.

1. Pick an arbitrary node (say node 1) of the original graph, and extract its connected component, $C(1)$.
2. If $|C(1)| \leq k_0$, pick a new node not contained in the previously extracted components.
3. If $\left||C(1)| - (1 - p_{\text{ext}}(\lambda))n\right| \leq \delta n$, stop the procedure, claiming a successful identification of the giant component.
4. If neither of the two conditions prevails, stop the procedure, admitting failure to identify the giant component.

In other words we repeatedly extract connected components, until either success (i.e. component of size L: $\left|L - (1 - p_{\text{ext}}(\lambda))n\right| \leq \delta n$) or failure (no success and a component of size $> k_0$) occurs, up to k times, for some k to be determined. After i extractions, which have been neither failures nor successes, we are left with an E-R graph with parameters n' and p, where

$$n' \in [n - ik_0, n - i],$$

since we have removed at most k_0 nodes and at least one node in each extraction. Thus at each step, Lemma 2.6 applies to the remaining graph, since for bounded k, the product $n'p$ remains close to λ.

Note that (a) by Lemma 2.5, the probability of finding a small component (of size at most k_0) is bounded above by $p_{\text{ext}}(\lambda) + \epsilon$, and (b) by Lemma 2.6, the probability of failure is bounded above by ϵ. Thus at each step, the probability of success is bounded below by $1 - p_{\text{ext}}(\lambda) - 2\epsilon$, so that

$$\mathbf{P}(\text{Success in at most } k \text{ steps}) \geq \sum_{i=1}^{k}(p_{\text{ext}}(\lambda) - \epsilon)^{i-1}(1 - p_{\text{ext}}(\lambda) - 2\epsilon)$$

$$= (1 - p_{\text{ext}}(\lambda) - 2\epsilon)\frac{1 - (p_{\text{ext}}(\lambda) - \epsilon)^k}{1 - p_{\text{ext}}(\lambda) + \epsilon} \; .$$

By choosing k such that $(p_{\text{ext}}(\lambda) - \epsilon)^k \leq \epsilon$, we ensure that this probability of success is at least $1 - O(\epsilon)$.

To conclude, conditional on success, we have one giant component of the right size, up to k components of size at most k_0, and the remaining graph is an E-R graph with n'' nodes, where

$$n'' \in [n(p_{\text{ext}}(\lambda) - \delta) - kk_0, n(p_{\text{ext}}(\lambda) + \delta)] \; .$$

Note now that the corresponding product $n''p$ is close to $p_{\text{ext}}(\lambda)\lambda$, i.e. the conjugate parameter of λ, as defined in Chapter 1, in the discussion of dual branching processes. Therefore, this remaining E-R graph is subcritical, and by the first half of Theorem 2.1 its largest component is of logarithmic size.

2.5 The critical regime

This section is the most advanced of the chapter, because it uses so-called martingales, which are defined below. Later chapters can be read independently of this section, the only part used subsequently being the definition of martingales.

We now consider the critical regime, where $\lambda = np = 1$, and establish bounds on the size of the largest connected component C_1. We first establish the following result.

Proposition 2.7 *For the random graph $G(n, 1/n)$, for n large enough, there is a constant $\kappa > 0$ such that for any node v,*

$$\mathbf{E}[|C(v)|] \leq \kappa n^{1/3} \; . \tag{2.9}$$

Proof Recall the recursion

$$A_{i+1} = A_i - 1 + \xi_{i+1} \tag{2.10}$$

for the number of active nodes in the exploration of the connected component $C(v)$, and the characterisation of $|C(v)|$ as

$$\tau := \min\{i \geq 1 : A_i = 0\}.$$

To prove the proposition, we use a coupling of the sequence $(A_i)_{i\geq 0}$ with a random walk with binomial increments. More precisely, we consider a sequence $(X_i)_{i\geq 1}$ of i.i.d. $\text{Bin}(n, 1/n)$ random variables, such that $\xi_i \leq X_i$ for all i.

Consider then the random walk $(S_i)_{i\geq 1}$, defined by $S_0 = 1$ and

$$S_i = S_{i-1} + X_i - 1 = 1 + \sum_{j=1}^{i}(X_j - 1), \ i \geq 1. \tag{2.11}$$

Fix $H > 0$ and define γ by

$$\gamma = \min\{i \geq 1, \ S_i \geq H \text{ or } S_i = 0\}.$$

It is readily seen by induction that $S_i \geq A_i$ for all $i \leq \gamma$. We now define the notion of a *martingale*.

Definition 2.8 (Martingale) A stochastic process $\{S_i\}_{i\geq 0}$ is a *martingale* if for all $i > 0$ the following identity holds:

$$\mathbf{E}(S_i \mid S_0, \ldots, S_{i-1}) = S_{i-1}. \tag{2.12}$$

This is an important notion, as many central results for sequences of i.i.d random variables (such as the law of large numbers or the central limit theorem) have natural extensions to martingales.

Obviously, the process $(S_i)_{i\geq 0}$ as defined in (2.11) is a martingale. Thus the optional stopping theorem (see e.g. [84]) gives

$$\mathbf{E}(S_0) = \mathbf{E}(S_\gamma) \geq H\mathbf{P}(S_\gamma \geq H).$$

Consequently, for $H > 0$,

$$\mathbf{P}(S_\gamma \geq H) \leq \frac{1}{H}. \tag{2.13}$$

We will now need the following result.

Lemma 2.9 *Let X be distributed according to $\text{Bin}(n, 1/n)$ and let f be an increasing function. Then*

$$\mathbf{E}[f(S_\gamma - H) \mid S_\gamma \geq H] \leq \mathbf{E}f(X). \tag{2.14}$$

Before proving the lemma we introduce the notion of stochastic order, or domination [72].

Definition 2.10 (Stochastic order, or domination) Let X and Y be two real-valued random variables with cumulative distribution functions F_X and F_Y respectively. We say that X is *stochastically dominated* by Y, written $X \leq_{\text{st}} Y$, if $F_X(t) \geq F_Y(t)$ for all real t, i.e. $\mathbf{P}(X \leq t) \geq \mathbf{P}(Y \leq t)$ for all real t.

Proof Let X be a random variable with $\text{Bin}(n, 1/n)$ distribution. We can write X as a sum of n Bernoulli independent random variables $(I_j)_{j=1,\ldots,n}$ with parameter $1/n$. Let J be the minimal index such that $\sum_{k=1}^{J} I_k = r + 1$, i.e.

$$J = \min\left\{ j \geq 1, \sum_{k=1}^{j} I_k = r + 1 \right\}.$$

Given J, the conditional distribution of $X - r + 1$ is $\text{Bin}(n - J, 1/n)$, which is obviously stochastically dominated by $\text{Bin}(n, 1/n)$. Let f be an increasing real function. Using the fact that $\{X \geq r + 1\} = \{J \leq n\}$, one obtains

$$\mathbf{E}[f(X - (r + 1)) \mid X \geq r + 1] = \frac{1}{\mathbf{P}(X \geq r + 1)} \, \mathbf{E}\left(f\left(\sum_{j=J+1}^{n} I_j \right) \mathbf{1}_{\{X \geq r+1\}} \right)$$

$$= \frac{1}{\mathbf{P}(J \leq n)} \, \mathbf{E}\left(\sum_{i=1}^{n} f\left(\sum_{j=i+1}^{n} I_j \right) \mathbf{1}_{\{J=i\}} \right)$$

$$\leq \frac{1}{\mathbf{P}(J \leq n)} \sum_{i=1}^{n} \mathbf{E}\left(f\left(\sum_{j=1}^{i} I_j' + \sum_{j=i+1}^{n} I_j \right) \mathbf{1}_{\{J=i\}} \right),$$

where $(I_j')_{j \geq 1}$ are i.i.d. Bernoulli random variables with parameter $1/n$, which are independent of $(I_j)_{j \geq 1}$. Therefore, by the independence between the I_j and the I_j', one has

$$\mathbf{E}[f(X - (r + 1)) \mid X \geq r + 1] \leq \frac{1}{\mathbf{P}(J \leq n)} \, \mathbf{E}\left(f\left(\sum_{j=1}^{n} I_j \right) \sum_{i=1}^{n} \mathbf{E}\left(\mathbf{1}_{\{J=i\}} \right) \right) = \mathbf{E}f(X).$$

Now consider $l \in \mathbb{N}$ and $r \in \{1, \ldots, H - 1\}$.
Given $\{\gamma = l\} \cap \{S_{\gamma-1} = H - r\}$, we have

$$\mathbf{E}[f(S_\gamma - H) \mid S_\gamma \geq H] = \mathbf{E}[f(X - (r + 1)) \mid X \geq r + 1]$$
$$\leq \mathbf{E}f(X).$$

The result follows by de-conditioning over l and r. $\qquad\square$

Apply (2.14) with $f(x) = 2Hx + x^2$ to obtain

$$\mathbf{E}[2H(S_\gamma - H) + (S_\gamma - H)^2 \mid S_\gamma \geq H] \leq \mathbf{E}[X^2 + 2HX]$$
$$= 1 + \frac{n-1}{n} + 2H$$
$$\leq 2H + 2.$$

Writing $S_\gamma^2 = H^2 + 2H(S_\gamma - H) + (S_\gamma - H)^2$, this inequality yields, for $H \geq 2$,

$$\mathbf{E}(S_\gamma^2 \mid S_\gamma \geq H) \leq H^2 + 2H + 2 \leq H^2 + 3H. \qquad (2.15)$$

Noting that $S_i^2 - (1 - \frac{1}{n})i$ is a martingale, one can apply the optional stopping theorem to obtain

$$\mathbf{E}\left[S_\gamma^2 - \left(1 - \frac{1}{n}\right)\gamma\right] = 1 .$$

Combined with (2.13) and (2.15), this yields

$$\left(1 - \frac{1}{n}\right)\mathbf{E}\gamma = \mathbf{E}(S_\gamma^2) - 1 = \mathbf{P}(S_\gamma \geq H)\mathbf{E}[S_\gamma^2 \mid S_\gamma \geq H] - 1 \leq H + 2 .$$

Hence, for $n \geq 2$,

$$\mathbf{E}\gamma \leq \frac{n}{n-1}(H+2) \leq 2H + 4 . \tag{2.16}$$

Let $\tau_0 = \min\{i \geq 0 : A_{\gamma+i} = 0\}$. First note that if $S_\gamma = 0$, then $\tau \leq \gamma$. Therefore $\tau \leq \gamma + \tau_0 \mathbf{1}_{\{S_\gamma \geq H\}}$, so that

$$\mathbf{E}\tau \leq \mathbf{E}\gamma + \mathbf{E}(\tau_0 \mid S_\gamma \geq H)\mathbf{P}(S_\gamma \geq H) . \tag{2.17}$$

Conditional on A_{i-1}, ξ_i is distributed according to $\mathrm{Bin}(n - A_{i-1} - i - 1, 1/n)$. We now choose to let ξ_i be distributed as $\mathrm{Bin}(n - i, 1/n)$ for $i \geq \tau$. This affects neither the distribution of τ nor the existence of the coupled random walk $\{S_j\}_{j \geq 0}$. With this modification, ξ_i is stochastically dominated by $\mathrm{Bin}(n-i, 1/n)$ for all $i \geq 0$, which implies that

$$\mathbf{E}(\xi_i - 1) \leq \frac{n-i}{n} - 1 = -\frac{i}{n} .$$

Thus the process $\eta_i := A_{\gamma+i} + \sum_{j=1}^{i} \frac{j}{n}$ is a supermartingale, i.e. a process where (2.12) holds with inequality sign $\leq$ instead of equality. By the optional stopping theorem, one has

$$\mathbf{E}(\eta_{\tau_0} \mid S_\gamma \geq H) \leq \mathbf{E}(\eta_0 \mid S_\gamma \geq H) = \mathbf{E}(A_\gamma \mid S_\gamma \geq H)$$
$$\leq \mathbf{E}(S_\gamma \mid S_\gamma \geq H)$$
$$\leq H + 1 ,$$

where the last inequality follows from Lemma 2.9. By the obvious inequality,

$$\eta_i \geq \sum_{j=1}^{i} \frac{j}{n} = \frac{i(i+1)}{2n} \geq \frac{i^2}{2n} ,$$

which implies

$$\frac{\mathbf{E}(\tau_0^2 \mid S_\gamma \geq H)}{2n} \leq H + 1 .$$

Now by Jensen's inequality, $(\mathbf{E}[\tau_0 \mathbf{1}_{\{S_\gamma \geq H\}}])^2 \leq \mathbf{E}[\tau_0^2 \mathbf{1}_{\{S_\gamma \geq H\}}]$. Hence,

$$\mathbf{E}(\tau_0 \mid S_\gamma \geq H) \leq \sqrt{2n(H+1)} . \tag{2.18}$$

Combined together, (2.13), (2.16), (2.17) and (2.18) yield

$$\mathbf{E}\tau \leq 2H + 4 + \frac{1}{H}\sqrt{2n(H+1)} \leq 2H + 2\sqrt{n/H} + 4 . \tag{2.19}$$

Take $H = (n/4)^{1/3}$ in (2.19). This yields the existence of a fixed positive $\kappa > 0$ such that for all positive n,

$$\mathbf{E}[|C(v)|] = \mathbf{E}\tau \leq \kappa n^{1/3} . \tag{2.20}$$

$\square$

Proof of Theorem 2.1 (iii) Let $(|C_j|)_{j\geq 1}$ denote the sizes of the connected components of $G(n, 1/n)$ ordered in decreasing order. By symmetry,

$$\mathbf{E}[|C(v)|] = \frac{1}{n}\mathbf{E}\left[\sum_{i=1}^{n}|C(i)|\right] = \frac{1}{n}\mathbf{E}\left[\sum_{j\geq 1}|C_j|^2\right] ,$$

where the second equality follows from the fact that in the middle term we count each C_j exactly $|C_j|$ times, for every $j \geq 1$. Thus, by (2.9),

$$\mathbf{E}\left[|C_1|^2\right] \leq \mathbf{E}\left[\sum_{j\geq 1}|C_j|^2\right] \leq \kappa n^{4/3} .$$

By Markov's inequality, one then has

$$\mathbf{P}(|C_1| \geq an^{2/3}) \leq \frac{\mathbf{E}[|C_1|^2]}{a^2 n^{4/3}} \leq \frac{\kappa}{a^2} ,$$

as stated.

2.6 Notes

A general introduction to epidemics and rumour models is presented in Bailey [5] and in Daley and Gani [23]. SIR models in which infectious periods have arbitrary probability distributions give rise to non-Markovian systems. For a detailed presentation of these models, see Andersson and Britton [3]. The connection between Reed–Frost epidemics and Erdős–Rényi random graphs was first described in Barbour and Mollison [10]. Galton–Watson processes are also instrumental in the study of more general families of random graphs (see Bollobás *et al.* [15]). The emergence of the giant component was first analysed in the seminal papers of Erdős and Rényi published from 1959 to 1961 [29], [30], [31]; see Bollobás [13] for a more complete set of references. The treatment given here is inspired by that in Alon and Spencer [2]. The upper bound on the size of the largest component in the critical regime, together with its proof, is taken from Peres [74]. One can consult Aldous [1] for an insightful analysis of the structure of connected components in this critical regime, and a characterisation of their sizes in terms of excursions of Brownian motions.

3

Connectivity and Poisson approximation

3.1 Introduction

In Chapter 2 we saw that, when the average degree np of an Erdős–Rényi graph is of constant order $\lambda > 1$, the graph contains a giant component of size of order n with high probability. However, in that regime, this component's size is strictly less than n, so that the graph is disconnected.

In the present chapter we shall establish that connectivity appears when the product np is of order $\log n$. We shall more precisely evaluate the probability of connectivity when np is asymptotic to $\log n + c$ for some constant c. In the framework of the Reed–Frost epidemic this corresponds to a regime known as *atomic infection* wherein all nodes are ultimately infected. In this regime we can analyse the time, in terms of the number of rounds, it takes the epidemic or the rumour to reach the whole population. This will be illustrated in Chapter 4 for the Reed–Frost epidemic and revisited in Chapter 6 when we introduce the small-world phenomenon.

The main mathematical tool required to prove the connectivity regime consists of Poisson approximation techniques, namely the *Stein–Chen method*. The Stein–Chen method provides bounds on how accurately a sum of $\{0, 1\}$-valued or Bernoulli random variables can be approximated by a Poisson distribution.

3.2 Variation distance

The Stein–Chen method provides bounds on the accuracy of Poisson approximation in terms of the variation distance, which we now introduce, together with some of its main properties.

Definition 3.1 (Variation distance)   The *variation distance* between two probability measures μ_1, μ_2 on the same measurable space $(\Omega, \mathcal{F})$ is defined as

$$d_{\text{var}}(\mu_1, \mu_2) = 2 \sup_{A \in \mathcal{F}} |\mu_1(A) - \mu_2(A)| \, .$$

This distance admits an alternative characterisation.

Proposition 3.2   *Let a measure μ be such that both μ_1 and μ_2 are absolutely continuous with respect to μ (by definition this means that for all $A \in \mathcal{F}$, $\mu_i(A) > 0 \Rightarrow \mu(A) > 0$; e.g. the measure $\mu = \mu_1 + \mu_2$ satisfies this). Then the variation distance satisfies*

$$d_{\text{var}}(\mu_1, \mu_2) = \int_{\Omega} \left| \frac{d\mu_1}{d\mu}(\omega) - \frac{d\mu_2}{d\mu}(\omega) \right| \mu(d\omega),$$

where $d\mu_i/d\mu$ is the Radon–Nikodym derivative (or density) of μ_i with respect to μ.

In particular, for μ_1 and μ_2 probability measures on $\mathbb{N}$,

$$d_{\text{var}}(\mu_1, \mu_2) = \sum_{n \in \mathbb{N}} |\mu_1(n) - \mu_2(n)|.$$

Proof   For any $A \in \mathcal{F}$, let $\bar{A}$ be its complement. We then have

$$2|\mu_1(A) - \mu_2(A)| = |\mu_1(A) - \mu_2(A)| + |\mu_2(\bar{A}) - \mu_1(\bar{A})|$$

$$= \left| \int_{\Omega} \mathbf{1}_A(\omega) \left[\frac{d\mu_1}{d\mu} - \frac{d\mu_2}{d\mu} \right] d\mu \right| + \left| \int_{\Omega} \mathbf{1}_{\bar{A}}(\omega) \left[\frac{d\mu_1}{d\mu} - \frac{d\mu_2}{d\mu} \right] d\mu \right|$$

$$\leq \int_{\Omega} \left| \frac{d\mu_1}{d\mu} - \frac{d\mu_2}{d\mu} \right| d\mu.$$

Conversely, defining

$$A = \left\{ \omega : \frac{d\mu_1}{d\mu}(\omega) > \frac{d\mu_2}{d\mu}(\omega) \right\},$$

one has

$$\int_{\Omega} \left| \frac{d\mu_1}{d\mu} - \frac{d\mu_2}{d\mu} \right| d\mu = \mu_1(A) - \mu_2(A) + \mu_2(\bar{A}) - \mu_1(\bar{A})$$

$$= 2|\mu_1(A) - \mu_2(A)|.$$

$\square$

The next proposition relates variation distance and weak convergence. We first define the notion of weak convergence of probability measures.

Definition 3.3 (Weak convergence)   A sequence of probability measures $\{\mu_n\}_{n\geq 0}$ is said to *converge weakly* to μ_∞ if, for all bounded and continuous functions f,

$$\lim_{n\to\infty} \int_\Omega f(\omega)\mu_n(d\omega) = \int_\Omega f(\omega)\mu_\infty(d\omega).$$

Proposition 3.4   *Assume that for a sequence of probability measures* $\{\mu_n\}_{n\geq 0}$, *there exists a probability measure* μ_∞ *such that*

$$\lim_{n\to\infty} d_{\mathrm{var}}(\mu_n, \mu_\infty) = 0.$$

Then μ_n *converges weakly to* μ_∞ *as* $n \to \infty$.

Proof   For any n and any bounded measurable function f,

$$\left| \int_\Omega f(\omega)\mu_n(d\omega) - \int_\Omega f(\omega)\mu_\infty(d\omega) \right| \leq \sup_{\omega\in\Omega}|f(\omega)|\, d_{\mathrm{var}}(\mu_n, \mu_\infty).$$

Indeed, this follows by writing, for some measure μ such that both μ_n and μ_∞ are absolutely continuous with respect to it

$$\left| \int_\Omega f(\omega)\mu_n(d\omega) - \int_\Omega f(\omega)\mu_\infty(d\omega) \right| \leq \int_\Omega |f(\omega)| \left| \frac{d\mu_n}{d\mu}(\omega) - \frac{d\mu_\infty}{d\mu}(\omega) \right| \mu(d\omega)$$

$$\leq \sup_{\omega\in\Omega}|f(\omega)|\, d_{\mathrm{var}}(\mu_n, \mu_\infty),$$

where we use the characterisation of variation distance given in Proposition 3.2. Thus convergence in variation implies weak convergence.   □

3.3 The Stein–Chen method

The Stein–Chen method is an explicit technique for obtaining an approximation of the distribution of an integer-valued random variable by a Poisson distribution. This is known as *Poisson approximation*.

Let V be a finite or countable set, and let $(I_j)_{j\in V}$ be a family of not necessarily independent Bernoulli random variables. Let $\pi_j := \mathbf{P}(I_j = 1)$, and let $\lambda := \sum_{j\in V} \pi_j$.

For an arbitrary subset $A \subset \mathbb{N}$, we are interested in evaluating the probability $\mathbf{P}(X \in A)$, where $X = \sum_{j\in V} I_j$. The Stein–Chen method enables us to bound the error made when approximating this probability by the corresponding probability

$$P_\lambda(A) := \sum_{k\in A} e^{-\lambda} \lambda^k / k!\,,$$

i.e. the probability that a Poisson random variable with parameter λ lies in A.

In fact, it provides bounds on the variation distance between the distribution of X and the Poisson distribution P_λ.

In what follows, we will denote by $\mathcal{L}(X)$ the law or distribution of the random variable X.

Theorem 3.5 *Assume that there exist random variables $(J_{ij})_{i,j \in V, j \neq i}$ defined on the same probability space as $(I_j)_{j \in V}$ and such that for all $i \in V$, the following equality of distributions holds:*

$$\mathcal{L}\big((J_{ij})_{j \in V, j \neq i}\big) = \mathcal{L}\big((I_j)_{j \in V, j \neq i} \,\big|\, I_i = 1\big).$$

Then

$$d_{\mathrm{var}}(\mathcal{L}(X), P_\lambda) \leq 2 \frac{1 - e^{-\lambda}}{\lambda} \sum_{i \in V} \pi_i \Big(\pi_i + \sum_{j \in V, j \neq i} \mathbf{E}\big|I_j - J_{ij}\big|\Big).$$

Remark 3.6 Note that the term $\lambda^{-1}(1 - \exp(-\lambda))$ in the previous inequality is no larger than $\min(1, \lambda)$. Theorem 3.5 is often used with this term instead.

Before we prove the theorem we need some preliminary results. For an arbitrary subset $A \subset \mathbb{N}$, define the function f_A by $f_A(0) = 0$, and for $i \in \mathbb{N}$,

$$f_A(i + 1) = \frac{P_\lambda(A \cap \{0, 1, \ldots, i\}) - P_\lambda(A)P_\lambda(\{0, 1, \ldots, i\})}{\lambda P_\lambda(\{i\})}. \tag{3.1}$$

It is easy to check that

$$\lambda f_A(i + 1) - i f_A(i) = \mathbf{1}_{\{i \in A\}} - P_\lambda(A).$$

Multiplying both sides by $\mathbf{P}(X = i)$ and summing over $i \in V$ yields

$$\mathbf{E}(\lambda f_A(X + 1) - X f_A(X)) = \mathbf{P}(X \in A) - P_\lambda(A). \tag{3.2}$$

We now need the following lemma.

Lemma 3.7 *The function f_A defined in (3.1) satisfies*

$$\sup_{i \geq 0}\big|f_A(i + 1) - f_A(i)\big| \leq \frac{1 - e^{-\lambda}}{\lambda}.$$

Proof Remark that

$$f_A(i + 1) - f_A(i) = \sum_{j \in A}(f_{\{j\}}(i + 1) - f_{\{j\}}(i)) \leq f_{\{i\}}(i + 1) - f_{\{i\}}(i),$$

where $f_{\{j\}}(.)$ is defined as f_A, for the particular set $A = \{j\}$. The inequality follows from the fact that $f_{\{i\}}(i + 1) - f_{\{i\}}(i)$ is the only positive term in the sum over A. This in turn holds by the following arguments.

From equation (3.1), for $j > i$, one has

$$f_{\{j\}}(i + 1) = -\frac{P_\lambda(\{j\})P_\lambda(\{0, \ldots, i\})}{\lambda P_\lambda(\{i\})} = -P_\lambda(\{j\}) \sum_{k=0}^{i} \binom{i}{k} \frac{k!}{\lambda^{k+1}},$$

which is clearly negative and decreasing in i.

Similarly, for $j < i$, one has

$$f_{\{j\}}(i + 1) = \frac{P_\lambda(\{j\})[1 - P_\lambda(\{0, \ldots, i\})]}{\lambda P_\lambda(\{i\})} = P_\lambda(\{j\}) \sum_{k=0}^{\infty} \frac{1}{\binom{k+i+1}{k+1}} \frac{\lambda^k}{(k + 1)!},$$

which is clearly positive and decreasing in i.

Hence, it follows that

$$
\begin{aligned}
f_A(i + 1) - f_A(i) &\le f_{\{i\}}(i + 1) - f_{\{i\}}(i) \\
&= \frac{P_\lambda(\{i\})[1 - P_\lambda(\{0, 1, \ldots, i\})]}{\lambda P_\lambda(\{i\})} + \frac{P_\lambda(\{i\})P_\lambda(\{0, 1, \ldots, i - 1\})}{\lambda P_\lambda(\{i - 1\})} \\
&= \frac{1}{\lambda}\left[1 - P_\lambda(\{0, 1, \ldots, i\}) + \frac{\lambda}{i}P_\lambda(\{0, 1, \ldots, i - 1\})\right] \\
&\le \frac{1}{\lambda}\left[1 - P_\lambda(\{0, 1, \ldots, i\}) + P_\lambda(\{1, 2, \ldots, i\})\right] \\
&= \frac{1 - P_\lambda(\{0\})}{\lambda} = \frac{1 - e^{-\lambda}}{\lambda}.
\end{aligned}
$$

Replacing A by its complement $\bar{A}$, and noting that $f_A(i) = -f_{\bar{A}}(i)$, we have by the same argument that

$$f_{\bar{A}}(i + 1) - f_{\bar{A}}(i) \le \frac{1 - e^{-\lambda}}{\lambda},$$

so that

$$f_A(i + 1) - f_A(i) \ge -\frac{1 - e^{-\lambda}}{\lambda}.$$

□

Proof of Theorem 3.5. We recast equality (3.2) as follows; to simplify notations, we denote f_A by f:

$$
\begin{aligned}
\mathbf{P}(X \in A) - P_\lambda(A) &= \mathbf{E}\big(\lambda f(X + 1) - X f(X)\big) \\
&= \sum_{i \in V} \pi_i \mathbf{E} f(X + 1) - \sum_{i \in V} \mathbf{E}\big(I_i f(X)\big) \\
&= \sum_{i \in V} \pi_i \mathbf{E} f(X + 1) - \sum_{i \in V} \mathbf{P}(I_i = 1)\mathbf{E}\big(f(X) \mid I_i = 1\big) \\
&= \sum_{i \in V} \pi_i \mathbf{E} f(X + 1) - \sum_{i \in V} \pi_i \mathbf{E}\big(f(\sum_{j \neq i} J_{ij} + 1)\big) \\
&= \sum_{i \in V} \pi_i \mathbf{E}\big(f(X + 1) - f(\sum_{j \neq i} J_{ij} + 1)\big).
\end{aligned}
$$

Using Lemma 3.7 and the triangular inequality, we have for all i and j

$$|f(i) - f(j)| \le |i - j|\frac{1 - e^{-\lambda}}{\lambda}.$$

Therefore,

$$\left|\mathbf{P}(X \in A) - P_\lambda(A)\right| \le \frac{1 - e^{-\lambda}}{\lambda} \sum_{i \in V} \pi_i \mathbf{E} \left| \sum_{j \in V} I_j - \sum_{j \neq i} J_{ij} \right|$$

$$\le \frac{1 - e^{-\lambda}}{\lambda} \sum_{i \in V} \pi_i \left(\pi_i + \sum_{j \neq i} \mathbf{E} \left| I_j - J_{ij} \right| \right).$$

We conclude using the fact that the total variation distance is given by

$$d_{\mathrm{var}}(\mathcal{L}(X), P_\lambda) = 2 \sup_{A \subset \mathbb{N}} \left| \mathbf{P}(X \in A) - P_\lambda(A) \right|.$$

$\square$

3.4 Emergence of connectivity in E-R graphs

To analyse connectivity of the random graph $G(n, p)$, we first evaluate the probability that there are no isolated nodes using Poisson approximation. We then show that, with high probability, disconnections are due to isolated nodes only.

3.4.1 The number of isolated nodes

Recall that the *degree* of a node is the number of its graph neighbours, and that a node is *isolated* if it has zero degree, i.e. no neighbours. Clearly, when the graph contains an isolated node, it cannot be connected. The study of the presence or not of isolated nodes will thus give us upper bounds on the probability that the graph is connected.

Let I_v equal 1 if node v is isolated, and 0 otherwise. Recalling that $\xi_{uv} \in \{0, 1\}$ indicates the presence of edge (u, v), it thus holds that

$$I_v = \prod_{w \neq v} \mathbf{1}_{\xi_{vw}=0} = \prod_{w \neq v} (1 - \xi_{vw}).$$

The number of isolated nodes is thus

$$X = \sum_{v=1}^n I_v.$$

We then have the following.

Theorem 3.8   *Assume that for some fixed $c \in \mathbb{R}$, $np = \log n + c$. Then the distribution of the number X of isolated nodes in $G(n, p)$ converges in variation, as $n \to \infty$, to the Poisson distribution with parameter e^{-c}.*

Proof We use the Stein–Chen method. Set

$$J_{vw} = \prod_{u \neq v, w} \mathbf{1}_{\xi_{uw}=0} = \prod_{u \neq v, w} (1 - \xi_{uw}), \quad v, w \in \{1, \ldots, n\}, \ w \neq v.$$

Note that conditioning on $I_v = 1$ is equivalent to conditioning on $\xi_{vw} = 0$ for all $w \neq v$.

Conditional on this event, all other edge indicator variables are left unaffected, by independence. We therefore have the equality of distributions

$$\mathcal{L}(\{J_{vw}\}_{w \neq v}) = \mathcal{L}(\{I_w\}_{w \neq v} \mid I_v = 1).$$

Let $\pi = \mathbf{E}(I_v) = (1 - p)^{n-1}$ and $\lambda = \mathbf{E}(X) = n\pi$. Applying Theorem 3.5, we have

$$d_{\mathrm{var}}(X, P_\lambda) \leq 2 \min(1, \lambda^{-1}) \, n\pi \left(\pi + \sum_{w=1, \, w \neq v}^{n} \mathbf{E}|I_w - J_{vw}| \right).$$

Note that

$$\mathbf{E}|I_w - J_{vw}| = \mathbf{E}\left(\xi_{vw} \prod_{u \neq v, w} (1 - \xi_{uw}) \right) = p(1 - p)^{n-2}.$$

This then yields

$$d_{\mathrm{var}}(X, P_\lambda) \leq 2 \min(1, \lambda^{-1}) \lambda [\pi + p(n - 1)\pi/(1 - p)] \leq 2 \left(\pi + \lambda \frac{p}{1 - p} \right).$$

By the evaluation

$$\lambda = n\pi = n \left(1 - \frac{\log(n) + c}{n} \right)^{n-1} \to e^{-c}$$

as $n \to \infty$, the upper bound is of order $(\log n)/n$ as $n \to \infty$. This establishes the convergence

$$\lim_{n \to \infty} d_{\mathrm{var}}(X, P_\lambda) = 0.$$

The triangle inequality further yields

$$d_{\mathrm{var}}(X, P_{e^{-c}}) \leq d_{\mathrm{var}}(P_{e^{-c}}, P_\lambda) + d_{\mathrm{var}}(X, P_\lambda).$$

It remains to show that $d_{\mathrm{var}}(P_{e^{-c}}, P_\lambda) \to 0$ as $n \to \infty$. This will follow from the next lemma. □

Lemma 3.9 *For $\lambda, \lambda' \geq 0$,*

$$d_{\mathrm{var}}(P_\lambda, P_{\lambda'}) \leq 2 \left(1 - e^{-|\lambda - \lambda'|} \right) \leq 2|\lambda - \lambda'|.$$

Proof Assume without loss of generality that $\lambda \geq \lambda'$. Let X, Y be two independent Poisson random variables with parameters λ', $\lambda - \lambda'$, respectively. Thus $X' := X + Y$ is Poisson with parameter λ. For any $A \subset \mathbb{N}$, write

$$
\begin{aligned}
2\big|&P_\lambda(A) - P_{\lambda'}(A)\big| \\
&= 2\big|\mathbf{P}(X + Y \in A) - \mathbf{P}(X \in A)\big| \\
&= 2\big|\mathbf{P}(Y = 0)\mathbf{P}(X \in A) - \mathbf{P}(X \in A) + \mathbf{P}(Y > 0, X + Y \in A)\big| \\
&\leq 2\mathbf{P}(Y > 0) .
\end{aligned}
$$

The upper bound that is given in the last line is independent of A and equal to $2(1 - e^{-|\lambda - \lambda'|})$. The result follows. $\qquad\square$

3.4.2 Probability of connectivity

We are now ready to establish the following result.

Theorem 3.10 *Let $c \in \mathbb{R}$ be given, and assume that p is such that $np = \log n + c$. One then has the limit*

$$
\lim_{n \to \infty} \mathbf{P}(G(n, p) \text{ connected}) = e^{-e^{-c}} . \tag{3.3}
$$

A direct consequence of this theorem is that if the average degree $(n - 1)p$ asymptotically dominates $\log n$, i.e. if c is replaced by c_n such that c_n tends to infinity as n increases, then the graph is connected with high probability, i.e. with a probability that tends to one as n goes to infinity.

Proof We first show that the probability that the graph contains connected components of sizes between 2 and $n/2$ goes to zero under the assumptions of the theorem. This will imply that the probability that the graph is connected is asymptotically equivalent to the probability that it has no isolated nodes. By Theorem 3.8, denoting by X the number of isolated nodes, it holds that

$$
\mathbf{P}(G(n, p) \text{ has no isolated nodes}) = \mathbf{P}(X = 0) \sim e^{-e^{-c}} ,
$$

hence the asserted result.

Let us first check that, with high probability, the graph has no connected components of size 2:

$$
\begin{aligned}
\mathbf{P}(&\exists \text{ connected component of size 2}) \\
&\leq \frac{n(n-1)}{2} \mathbf{P}((u, v) \text{ connected component of } G(n, p)) \\
&= \frac{n(n-1)}{2} p(1 - p)^{2(n-2)} .
\end{aligned}
$$

By the inequality $1 - x \le e^{-x}$ for $x \ge 0$, this expression is no larger than

$$n^2 \frac{p}{(1-p)^4} e^{-2np} .$$

This term is of order $p \sim (\log n)/n$, and thus asymptotically negligible.

We now show that the probability of having a connected component of size between 3 and $n/2$ vanishes asymptotically. To this end, we shall rely on Cayley's theorem according to which the number of trees on a set of r labelled nodes is exactly r^{r-2}.

For any $r \in \{3, \ldots, n/2\}$ and an arbitrary set C of r nodes, the probability that this set is a connected component of $G(n, p)$ is then no larger than

$$\sum_{\mathcal{T}} \mathbf{P}(\text{edges in } \mathcal{T} \text{ present and no edge between } C \text{ and } \bar{C})$$

$$\le r^{r-2} p^{r-1} (1-p)^{r(n-r)}, \quad (3.4)$$

where the sum is over all trees $\mathcal{T}$ on C.

Summing over all $r \in \{3, \ldots, n/2\}$ and all size-r components C, one obtains the following upper bound on the probability Π that there is a connected component of such size in $G(n, p)$:

$$\Pi \le \sum_{r=3}^{\lceil n/2 \rceil} \binom{n}{r} r^{r-2} p^{r-1} (1-p)^{r(n-r)} .$$

Using $\binom{n}{r} \le n^r/r!$ and Stirling's formula $r! \sim \sqrt{2\pi r}(r/e)^r$, one obtains

$$\Pi \le \sum_{r=3}^{\lceil n/2 \rceil} n^r \frac{1}{\sqrt{r}} \left[\left(\frac{e}{r}\right)^r r^{r-2} p^{r-1} e^{-pr(n-r)} \right] .$$

The inequality holds because the omission of the factor $1/\sqrt{2\pi}$ in the application of Stirling's formula more than compensates for the approximation made by replacing $1/r!$ by the formula.

After simplifying and using the fact that $n - r \ge n/2$ for r in the summation range, we obtain

$$\Pi \le \frac{1}{p} \sum_{r=3}^{\lceil n/2 \rceil} r^{-5/2} e^{r\{1 + \log np - (1/2)np\}} .$$

The exponent in curly brackets is equivalent to $-(1/2)np$; also, $1/p \le n$. Thus, for all $\epsilon > 0$, one has

$$\Pi \leq n \sum_{r=3}^{\lceil n/2 \rceil} r^{-5/2} e^{-r(1/2-\epsilon)np}$$

$$\leq n \sum_{r \geq 3} e^{-r(1/2-\epsilon)np}$$

$$= n \frac{e^{-3(1/2-\epsilon)np}}{1 - e^{-(1/2-\epsilon)np}}$$

$$= O(n^{-1/2+3\epsilon}),$$

which concludes the proof of the theorem. □

3.4.3 Cayley's theorem

We now show that the number of trees on a set $\{0, \ldots, r-1\}$ is r^{r-2}; this is the statement of Cayley's theorem. To this end we construct a bijection between sequences of $r - 2$ integers in $\{0, \ldots, r-1\}$ and the set of trees on this set.

Given a tree $\mathcal{T}$, one determines its associated *Prüfer sequence* or *Prüfer code* $\phi(\mathcal{T}) = \{w_1, \ldots, w_{r-2}\}$ as follows. By convention, node 0 is the root of the tree. The degree 1 nodes distinct from the root are called the "leaves" of the tree. One starts by picking the leaf with the smallest label, say v_1, and let w_1 be the label of the node v_1 it attaches to. One then examines the leaves of the reduced tree $\mathcal{T} \setminus \{v_1\}$, picks its smallest leaf, say v_2, and then w_2 is the label of the neighbour of v_2 in $\mathcal{T} \setminus \{v_1\}$. One repeats this procedure until only one leaf remains, i.e. after having extracted $r - 2$ labels.

To show that the function ϕ is bijective, let us see how the tree $\mathcal{T}$ is determined by $\phi(\mathcal{T})$. The first leaf v_1 that has been removed must be the smallest integer in $\{1, \ldots, r-1\}$ which does not appear in the sequence $\phi(\mathcal{T}) = \{w_1, \ldots, w_{r-2}\}$. One can thus reconstruct the edge (v_1, w_1). Similarly, the node removed next, v_2, is the smallest integer in $\{1, \ldots, r-1\} \setminus \{v_1\}$ which does not appear in $\{w_2, \ldots, w_{r-2}\}$, and we can thus reconstruct the edge (v_2, w_2). Iterating, we next reconstruct $(v_3, w_3), \ldots, (v_{r-2}, w_{r-2})$. There only remains one element in $\{1, \ldots, r-1\} \setminus \{v_1, \ldots, v_{r-2}\}$, say v_{r-1}. Necessarily, this last element is connected to the root 0, hence the edge $(v_{r-1}, 0)$ is also in tree $\mathcal{T}$. We have thus reconstructed the $r - 1$ edges of the tree $\mathcal{T}$.

3.5 Notes

The Stein–Chen method was introduced by Stein in 1972 as a method for bounding the distance of a random variable from the Normal distribution.

Later, in 1975, Chen showed that this method is not restricted to a normal limit and generalised the technique to Poisson distributions. More recently it has been applied to stochastic processes such as Poisson processes and diffusions; see Barbour *et al.* [9] for a complete set of references. The treatment given here is inspired by that of Lindvall [58].

The Stein–Chen method has been used to study a number of mathematical problems with applications in computer science, including the matching problem, the coupon collector problem and the birthday problem. We refer to Chatterjee *et al.* [18] for a rigorous treatment of these problems and to Mitzenmacher and Upfal [67] for details about how such problems arise in computer networks. For more details on the bijection between labelled trees and their Prüfer codes, see Lovász and Vesztergombi [60].

4

Diameter of Erdős–Rényi graphs

4.1 Introduction

Given a graph G, and two vertices u, v, the graph distance $d_G(u, v)$ is by definition the minimal length (in number of hops) of a path connecting u to v. The diameter of the graph G is then defined as the supremum over pairs of nodes u, v of the distance $d_G(u, v)$. It is denoted by $D(G)$:

$$D(G) = \sup_{\text{nodes } u,v} d_G(u, v).$$

Recall that an E-R graph captures the dynamics of a Reed–Frost epidemic started at a source node u, with $\Gamma_t(u) := \{v : d_G(u, v) = t\}$ representing the set of infectious nodes after t time steps. The epidemic will infect all nodes if and only if the graph is connected, which is equivalent to the diameter being finite. In that case, the diameter provides an upper bound on the time it takes for a Reed–Frost epidemic to reach all nodes.

The diameter of a graph is also interesting when the graph represents a network over which goods (such as information) need to be transported: it then gives an upper bound on the time for goods to travel from any location u to any other location v, provided shortest paths between locations are used.

The following result illustrates an interesting relation between the diameter, the number of nodes and the maximal node degree of a graph. In fact, given the maximal degree of the graph and its number of nodes, we derive a lower bound on the graph distance between any pair of nodes and thus on the diameter of the graph.

Lemma 4.1 *Given a graph G on n nodes, such that the maximal node degree is at most Δ ($\Delta > 2$), its diameter D satisfies*

$$n \le 1 + \Delta \frac{(\Delta - 1)^D - 1}{\Delta - 2}.$$

Equivalently, one has

$$D \geq \frac{\log\left(n\left[1 - \frac{2}{\Delta}\right] + \frac{2}{\Delta}\right)}{\log(\Delta - 1)}.$$

Proof Introduce the notation $d_i(u) = |\Gamma_i(u)|$. It is easily seen that, when the maximal node degree is at most Δ, for any u, $d_1(u) \leq \Delta$, and for all $i \geq 2$, $d_i(u) \leq \Delta(\Delta - 1)^{i-1}$. If the diameter is not larger than D, then necessarily

$$n = 1 + d_1(u) + \cdots + d_D(u) \leq 1 + \Delta\left\{1 + (\Delta - 1) + \cdots + (\Delta - 1)^{D-1}\right\}.$$

The result follows. □

It is not obvious a priori that this bound is tight. To show that it is fairly tight, we introduce the family of so-called *de Bruijn graphs*. One additional reason for examining these graphs is that they exhibit an interesting property, namely that "routing" can be done efficiently, as we explain below.

For two integers k, ℓ, the de Bruijn graph $B(k, \ell)$ has $n = k^\ell$ nodes, which are identified with the ℓ-letter words on the alphabet $\{1, \ldots, k\}$. A node $x_1 \ldots x_\ell$ is connected to nodes $yx_1 \ldots x_{\ell-1}$ and $x_2 \ldots x_\ell y$ for all $y \in \{1, \ldots, k\}$. Thus its degree is at most $\Delta = 2k$. Between any two nodes $x_1 \ldots x_\ell, y_1 \ldots y_\ell$ there is an ℓ-hop path, going through $x_2 \ldots x_\ell y_1$, $x_3 \ldots x_\ell y_1 y_2$, $\ldots$, $x_\ell y_1 \ldots y_{\ell-1}$.

Thus for the de Bruijn graph $B(k, \ell)$, the diameter is bounded as

$$D \leq \ell = \frac{\log n}{\log k} = \frac{\log n}{\log \Delta - \log 2}.$$

Let us now interpret the evaluation of the graph diameter in terms of routing. Routing consists of relaying a message along the graph edges to a destination node. Ideally, each local routing decision, i.e. the choice of next node to which to forward the message, should be based on minimal information. The evaluation above suggests the following routing algorithm, which requires only knowledge of the identity of the current node and that of the destination node. When at node $z = z_1 \ldots z_\ell$, a message with destination $y = y_1 \ldots y_\ell \neq z$ is processed as follows. First, determine the largest index $k < \ell$ such that $z_{\ell-k+1} \ldots z_\ell = y_1 \ldots y_k$. Then, forward the message to the next-hop node labelled $z_2 \ldots z_\ell y_{k+1}$. Clearly, such routing reaches the destination in at most ℓ hops, for any initial and final nodes.

For efficient routing to be possible, it is a prerequisite that the graph at hand have a small diameter; as we shall see in Chapter 6 on small worlds, it is by no means a sufficient condition. Let us now return to E-R graphs, and establish that they have diameter close to optimal, given their maximal degree and number of nodes.

4.2 Diameter of E-R graphs

In what follows we show that E-R graphs with average degree larger than $\log n$ have diameters that concentrate on only a finite number of values around $\frac{\log n}{2 \log \lambda}$, where $\lambda = np$. More precisely, let $\delta = (n - 1)p$ be the average node degree of $G(n, p)$, which is asymptotically equivalent, for n large, to λ. Then the following holds.

Theorem 4.2   *Assume that, for n large,*

$$\log n \ll \delta \ll \sqrt{n}. \tag{4.1}$$

Letting

$$D' = \left\lceil \frac{\log n}{2 \log \delta} \right\rceil, \tag{4.2}$$

it holds that

$$\lim_{n \to \infty} \mathbf{P}\left(D(G(n, p)) \in \{2D' - 3, 2D' - 2, 2D' - 1, 2D', 2D' + 1\}\right) = 1.$$

Using the fact that $x - 1 < \lceil x \rceil \le x$, the theorem asserts that the diameter of $G(n, p)$ takes with high probability at most five distinct values falling between

$$\left\lceil \frac{\log n}{\log \lambda} \right\rceil - 4 \quad and \quad \left\lceil \frac{\log n}{\log \lambda} \right\rceil + 1.$$

Remark 4.3   The best possible result, given in Bollobás [13], establishes that, in fact, $D(G(n, p))$ can take at most two values and identifies the probability of each value occurring.

The rest of the chapter gives the details of the proof of Theorem 4.2, proceeding as follows.

In Section 4.3 we prove a key lemma. It gives upper and lower bounds d_i^+ and d_i^- on the size of the set $\Gamma_i(u)$ of nodes at a distance i from node u.

In Section 4.4.1, we leverage the control we have on the size of the sets $\Gamma_i(u)$ and $\Gamma_i(v)$ for any two nodes u and v to show that the probability that there is no link between $\Gamma_{D'}(u)$ and $\Gamma_{D'}(v)$ goes to 0 as n goes to infinity. This enables us to conclude that the diameter $D(G(n, p))$ of $G(n, p)$ is at most $2D' + 1$ with high probability.

Finally, to prove a lower bound we combine the property of the growth of the size of the sets $\Gamma_i(u)$ with the fact that the intersection of $\Gamma_C(u)$ and $\Gamma_C(v)$, for two nodes u and v and $C = D' - 2$, is empty with high probability. This shows that the diameter $D(G(n, p))$ of $G(n, p)$ is at least $2D' - 3$ with high probability.

4.3 Control of neighbourhood growth

Given some $\epsilon > 0$, define the quantities

$$d_j^\pm = \begin{cases} (1 \pm \epsilon)^j \delta^j & \text{if } j = 1, 2, \\ (1 \pm \epsilon)^2 (1 \pm \frac{\epsilon}{\delta})^{j-2} \delta^j & \text{if } j = 3, \ldots, D'. \end{cases} \tag{4.3}$$

The key ingredient in the proof of Theorem 4.2 is the following lemma.

Lemma 4.4 *Let $\epsilon > 0$ be fixed. Define for all $u \in \{1, \ldots, n\}$ and all $i = 1, \ldots, D'$, the event $\mathcal{E}_i(u)$ by*

$$\mathcal{E}_i(u) = \{d_i^- \le d_i(u) \le d_i^+\}.$$

Assume condition (4.1) holds. Then for any fixed $K > 0$, for large enough n,

$$\mathbf{P}(\mathcal{E}_i(u)) \ge 1 - D' n^{-K}, \quad u \in \{1, \ldots, n\}, \ i = 1, \ldots, D'. \tag{4.4}$$

Proof Let $u \in \{1, \ldots, n\}$ and $i \in \{1, \ldots, D'\}$ be fixed. Note that, conditional on $d_1(u), \ldots, d_{i-1}(u)$, $d_i(u)$ admits a binomial distribution with parameters

$$\mathcal{L}(d_i(u) \mid d_1(u), \ldots, d_{i-1}(u))$$
$$= \text{Bin}\left(n - 1 - d_1(u) - \cdots - d_{i-1}(u), 1 - (1-p)^{d_{i-1}(u)}\right),$$

where $\mathcal{L}(X \mid \mathcal{F})$ is the law or distribution of the random variable X conditional on the event $\mathcal{F}$. Denote by $\bar{\mathcal{E}}_i(u)$ the complement of $\mathcal{E}_i(u)$. It readily follows that

$$\mathbf{P}(\bar{\mathcal{E}}_i(u) \mid \mathcal{E}_1(u), \ldots, \mathcal{E}_{i-1}(u))$$
$$\le \mathbf{P}\left(\text{Bin}(n, 1 - (1-p)^{d_{i-1}^+}) \ge d_i^+\right) \tag{4.5}$$
$$+ \mathbf{P}\left(\text{Bin}(n - 1 - d_1^+ - \cdots - d_{i-1}^+, 1 - (1-p)^{d_{i-1}^-}) \le d_i^-\right).$$

Note that, for all $j < D'$, one has

$$\begin{aligned} d_j^- \le d_j^+ \le d_{D'-1}^+ &\le \left(\frac{\delta(1+\epsilon)}{\delta + \epsilon}\right)^2 (\delta + \epsilon)^{(\log n)/(2 \log \delta)} \\ &\le \left(\frac{\delta(1+\epsilon)}{\delta + \epsilon}\right)^2 \exp\left(\frac{\log n}{2} \frac{\log(\delta + \epsilon)}{\log \delta}\right) \\ &\le \left(\frac{\delta(1+\epsilon)}{\delta + \epsilon}\right)^2 \sqrt{n} \exp\left(\frac{\log n}{2} \frac{\log(\delta + \epsilon) - \log \delta}{\log \delta}\right) \\ &\le \left(\frac{\delta(1+\epsilon)}{\delta + \epsilon}\right)^2 \sqrt{n} \exp\left(\frac{\epsilon \log n}{2\delta \log \delta}\right) \\ &= O(\sqrt{n}), \end{aligned} \tag{4.6}$$

where we use the fact that $\log(1+x) \le x$ for $x \ge 0$ and in view of the assumption that $\delta \gg \log n$. This can be used to establish the following estimates as $n \to \infty$:

$$n(1 - (1 - p)^{d^+_{i-1}}) = (1 + o(1))\delta d^+_{i-1},$$

$$(n - 1 - d^+_1 - \cdots - d^+_{i-1})(1 - (1 - p)^{d^-_{i-1}}) = (1 + o(1))\delta d^-_{i-1},$$

where the $o(1)$ term can be chosen independently of $i \le D'$. Indeed, the term $1 - (1 - p)^{d^\pm_{i-1}}$ also reads

$$
\begin{aligned}
1 - \exp\left(-pd^\pm_{i-1} + O(p^2 d^\pm_{i-1})\right) &= pd^\pm_{i-1} + O\left((pd^\pm_{i-1})^2\right) \\
&= pd^\pm_{i-1}\left(1 + O(pd^\pm_{i-1})\right) \\
&= pd^\pm_{i-1}\left(1 + O(\delta/\sqrt{n})\right),
\end{aligned}
$$

and the latter term is $o(1)$ since we assumed $\delta = o(\sqrt{n})$.

Furthermore, by (4.6), the term $n - 1 - d^+_1 - \cdots - d^+_{i-1}$ is larger than $n - D'O(\sqrt{n}) = n - O(\sqrt{n}\log n)$, and thus equals $n(1 + o(1))$.

The Chernoff bound of Lemma 2.4 for sums of independent $\{0, 1\}$-valued random variables, applied to the right-hand side of (4.5), thus yields

$$\mathbf{P}(\bar{\mathcal{E}}_i(u) \mid \mathcal{E}_1(u), \ldots, \mathcal{E}_{i-1}(u)) \le e^{-(1+o(1))\delta d^-_{i-1}h(-\epsilon_i)} + e^{-(1+o(1))\delta d^+_{i-1}h(\epsilon_i)}, \quad (4.7)$$

where $h(x) = (1 + x)\log(1 + x) - x$, and

$$\epsilon_i = \frac{d^+_i}{\delta d^+_{i-1}} - 1 = 1 - \frac{d^-_i}{\delta d^-_{i-1}}$$

and is given by ϵ for $i = 1, 2$, and by ϵ/δ for $i > 2$.

For $i = 1$ or 2, the exponents on the right-hand side of (4.7) are larger than $c\delta$ for some constant $c > 0$. Since we have assumed that $\delta \gg \log n$, for any fixed $K > 0$, the right-hand side of (4.7) is, in this case, less than n^{-K} for n large enough.

For $i > 2$, using the fact that $h(x) = (1 + o(x))x^2/2$, the exponents on the right-hand side of (4.7) are in this case larger than $c\delta d^\pm_{i-1}\delta^{-2}$ for some constant $c > 0$, and thus again of order at least δ. Thus for $i > 2$ as well, for any fixed $K > 0$, the right-hand side of (4.7) is less than n^{-K} for n large enough.

The claim of the lemma is finally established by writing

$$
\begin{aligned}
\mathbf{P}(\mathcal{E}_i(u)) &\ge \mathbf{P}(\mathcal{E}_1(u), \ldots, \mathcal{E}_i(u)) \\
&\ge \mathbf{P}(\mathcal{E}_1(u), \ldots, \mathcal{E}_{i-1}(u)) - \mathbf{P}(\bar{\mathcal{E}}_i(u) \mid \mathcal{E}_1(u), \ldots, \mathcal{E}_{i-1}(u)) \\
&\ge 1 - \sum_{j=1}^{i} \mathbf{P}(\bar{\mathcal{E}}_j(u) \mid \mathcal{E}_1(u), \ldots, \mathcal{E}_{j-1}(u)) \\
&\ge 1 - D'n^{-K}
\end{aligned}
$$

for n large enough. The result follows. $\qquad\square$

4.4 Bounds for the diameter

4.4.1 The upper bound

Let us first establish that, with high probability, $D(G(n, p)) \le 2D' + 1$. For two arbitrary nodes u, v, note that

$$\mathbf{P}(d_G(u, v) > 2D' + 1 \mid \Gamma_1(u), \dots, \Gamma_{D'}(u), \Gamma_1(v), \dots, \Gamma_{D'}(v)) \le (1 - p)^{d_{D'}(u)d_{D'}(v)} .$$

Indeed, given the neighbourhoods $\Gamma_i(u), \Gamma_i(v)$ for $i = 1, \dots, D'$, either they have nonempty intersection, in which case $d_G(u, v) \le 2D'$, or they do not intersect, in which case all of the $d_{D'}(u)d_{D'}(v)$ edges must be absent for $d_G(u, v) > 2D' + 1$ to hold. We thus obtain

$$\mathbf{P}(d_G(u, v) > 2D' + 1) \le \mathbf{P}(\bar{\mathcal{E}}_{D'}(u)) + \mathbf{P}(\bar{\mathcal{E}}_{D'}(v)) + (1 - p)^{2(d_{D'}^-)^2} .$$

The last term on the right-hand side is evaluated as follows:

$$
\begin{aligned}
(1 - p)^{2(d_{D'}^-)^2} &\le \exp\left(-2p\left[\frac{1 - \epsilon}{1 - \epsilon/\delta}\right]^4 (\delta - \epsilon)^{(\log n)/(\log \delta)}\right) \\
&\le \exp\left(-\eta p n^{1 - \epsilon/(\delta \log \delta)(1 + o(1))}\right) \\
&\le \exp(-\delta \eta)
\end{aligned}
$$

for some constant $\eta > 0$.

Since $\delta \gg \log n$, combined with Lemma 4.4, we find that for all $K > 0$, and sufficiently large n,

$$\mathbf{P}(d_G(u, v) > 2D' + 1) \le n^{-K} .$$

Finally,

$$\mathbf{P}(D(G(n, p)) > 2D' + 1) \le \sum_{u \ne v} \mathbf{P}(d_G(u, v) > 2D' + 1) \le n^2 \times n^{-K} .$$

By choosing $K > 2$, the desired upper bound is obtained.

4.4.2 The lower bound

The proof of the lower bound relies on the following lemma.

Lemma 4.5 *Given a set of n items, and two subsets C_1, C_2 both of size $r = o(\sqrt{n})$, selected independently and uniformly at random from sets of that size, it holds that*

$$\mathbf{P}(C_1 \cap C_2 = \emptyset) = (1 + o(1)) \exp\left(-\frac{r^2}{n} + O(r^3/(n - 2r)^2)\right)$$

and consequently that

$$\mathbf{P}(C_1 \cap C_2 \neq \emptyset) = O\!\left(\frac{r^2}{n}\right).$$

Proof   The probability that the intersection is empty equals

$$\frac{\binom{n-r}{r}}{\binom{n}{r}} = \frac{(n-r)!(n-r)!}{n!(n-2r)!}.$$

Stirling's formula yields the following equivalent:

$$\mathbf{P}(C_1 \cap C_2 = \emptyset) = (1 + o(1))\exp[(n-2r)\log(1 + r/(n-2r)) + n\log(1 - r/n)],$$

hence the result.   □

Let $C = D' - 2$. Conditioning on the neighbourhood sizes $d_1(u), \ldots, d_C(u)$, $d_1(v), \ldots, d_C(v)$, we have that

$$\mathbf{P}(d_G(u,v) \leq 2C \mid d_1(u), \ldots, d_C(u), d_1(v), \ldots, d_C(v)) \leq \mathbf{P}(C_1 \cap C_2 \neq \emptyset),$$

where C_1 and C_2 are sampled as in the previous lemma from an n-item set and have sizes

$$|C_1| = 1 + d_1(u) + \cdots + d_C(u), \quad |C_2| = 1 + d_1(v) + \cdots + d_C(v),$$

so that C_1 and C_2 are of size smaller than $1 + d_1^+ + \cdots + d_C^+$ with high probability, by Lemma 4.4. Moreover, a simple calculation yields

$$1 + d_1^+ + \cdots + d_C^+ = o(d_{D'-1}^+) = o(\sqrt{n}), \tag{4.8}$$

as $d_{D'-1}^+ = O(\sqrt{n})$ by (4.6).

Indeed, we may construct the successive neighbourhoods for the two nodes u, v as follows. First determine $\Gamma_1(u), \ldots, \Gamma_C(u)$. Let $\mathcal{N}'$ be the set of nodes not in any of these neighbourhoods. Conditional on these neighbourhoods, there are no edges between $\Gamma_i(u)$ and $\mathcal{N}'$ for all $i = 1, \ldots, C - 1$; the distribution of the edges internal to $\mathcal{N}'$ and between $\mathcal{N}'$ and $\Gamma_C(u)$ is unaffected by the conditioning. For convenience, we also introduce the notation $\mathcal{N}'' := \mathcal{N}' \cup \Gamma_C(u)$ and $\mathcal{B}_k(v) = \cup_{0 \leq i \leq k}\Gamma_i(v)$.

Now pick v at random from the total node set. If it falls in $\mathcal{N}'$, construct its first neighbourhood $\Gamma_1(v)$ by picking at random a set of size $d_1(v)$ from $\mathcal{N}'' \setminus \{v\}$. If this does not intersect $\Gamma_C(v)$, choose $\Gamma_2(v)$ as a random set of size $d_2(v)$ taken from $\mathcal{N}'' \setminus \mathcal{B}_1(v)$. Proceed until either all C neighbourhoods are constructed, or one does intersect $\Gamma_C(v)$.

The probability that this stopping condition occurs is given by the probability of intersection of two independently, randomly selected sets of sizes $|\mathcal{B}_C(u)|$ and $|\mathcal{B}_C(v)|$, respectively.

To conclude, by Lemmas 4.4 and 4.5, it holds that

$$\mathbf{P}(d_G(u, v) \le 2C)$$
$$= \mathbf{P}\left(d_G(u, v) \le 2C \mid \bigcap_{i=1}^C (\mathcal{E}_i(u) \cap \mathcal{E}_i(v))\right) \mathbf{P}\left(\bigcap_{i=1}^C (\mathcal{E}_i(u) \cap \mathcal{E}_i(v))\right)$$
$$+ \mathbf{P}\left(d_G(u, v) \le 2C \mid \bigcup_{i=1}^C \left(\bar{\mathcal{E}}_i(u) \cup \bar{\mathcal{E}}_i(v)\right)\right) \mathbf{P}\left(\bigcup_{i=1}^C \left(\bar{\mathcal{E}}_i(u) \cup \bar{\mathcal{E}}_i(v)\right)\right)$$
$$\le \mathbf{P}\left(d_G(u, v) \le 2C \mid \bigcap_{i=1}^C (\mathcal{E}_i(u) \cap \mathcal{E}_i(v))\right) + \mathbf{P}\left(\bigcup_{i=1}^C \left(\bar{\mathcal{E}}_i(u) \cup \bar{\mathcal{E}}_i(v)\right)\right)$$
$$\le \sum_{i=1}^C \left[\mathbf{P}(\bar{\mathcal{E}}_i(u)) + \mathbf{P}(\bar{\mathcal{E}}_i(v))\right] + O\left(\frac{(1 + d_1^+ + \ldots + d_C^+)^2}{n}\right)$$
$$\le 2D'n^{-K} + o(1),$$

where we have used (4.8) in the last step. Thus the right-hand side in the last line goes to zero as $n \to \infty$.

4.5 Notes

This chapter is based on the treatment by Bollobás, in Chapter 10 of [13], which contains a sharp analysis of the values that the diameter can take and the corresponding probabilities. Graphs achieving the bound of Lemma 4.1 are known as Moore graphs. We again direct the reader to [13], Chapter 10, for more information on the parameter values for which such graphs are known to exist.

5

From microscopic to macroscopic dynamics

5.1 Introduction

So far we have dealt with microscopic models of interaction and epidemic propagation. If we are interested in macroscopic characteristics, such as the time before a given fraction of the population is infected, a simpler analysis is often possible in which we can identify deterministic dynamic models, specified by differential equations, that reflect accurately the dynamics of the original system at a macroscopic level. Such macroscopic description is referred to as *mean-field approximation*.

Differential equations (macroscopic models) and Markov processes (microscopic models) are the basic models of dynamical systems in deterministic and probabilistic contexts, respectively. Since the analysis, both mathematical and computational, of differential equations is often more feasible and efficient, it is of interest to understand in some generality when the sample paths of a Markov process can be guaranteed to lie, with high probability, close to the solution of a differential equation.

We shall provide generic results applicable to all such contexts. In what follows we approximate certain families of jump processes depending on a parameter n usually interpreted as the total population size, and we approximate certain jump Markov processes as the parameter n becomes large. It is worth mentioning that the techniques presented here can be applied to a wide range of problems such as epidemic models, models for chemical reactions and population genetics, as well as other processes. More precisely the states of these systems can be normalised and interpreted as measuring population densities.

5.2 Birth and death processes

Suppose that we have a population of individuals belonging to d different species, where $X_i(t)$, $i = 1, \ldots, d$ is the total number of individuals of species i at time t. The process $X(t) = (X_i(t))_{i=1,\ldots,d}$ is assumed to be a Markov jump process on $\mathbb{N}^d$. That is to say, for any given pair of states $x, y \in \mathbb{N}^d$, the process jumps from state x to state y upon expiration of a random timer with exponential distribution, whose parameter depends on the pair of states (x, y). Such jumps can be interpreted as the compounding of deaths, births and mutations of individuals.

We suppose further that there is a finite number of possible jump directions $(e_i)_{i=1,\ldots,k}$ whose entries are restricted to belong to $\{-1, 0, 1\}$. We call such processes *birth and death processes*.

We shall denote by $\lambda_i(x)$ the rate at which transition from state x to state $x + e_i$ occurs.

Example 5.1 **The Poisson process:** *The Poisson process is the simplest non-trivial example of a birth and death process. It involves one type of individual, so the state space is $\mathbb{N}$, and the only transitions are births, with constant birth rate $\lambda(x) \equiv \lambda$ for all $x \in \mathbb{N}$, also called the intensity of the process. Denote by $N(t)$ the state at time t, starting with $N(0) = 0$. We recall here without proof some basic properties of the process:*

- *For all $s, t \in \mathbb{R}$, $N(t + s) - N(s)$ has the same distribution as $N(t)$, i.e. the Poisson distribution with parameter λt.*
- *For $s, t \in \mathbb{R}$, the random variable $N(t + s) - N(s)$ is independent of the past of the process before time s, i.e. $\{N(u)\}_{u \in [0,s]}$.*

The classical law of large numbers guarantees that for any fixed t, the ratio $(1/n)N(tn)$, being distributed as the sum of n i.i.d. Poisson random variables with parameter λt, converges almost surely to λt.

We now establish a functional version of this result, which will be the template for the main result of this chapter, namely Kurtz's theorem. It will also be the main ingredient in its proof.

Proposition 5.2 *Let N be a unit-rate Poisson process. Then for any $\epsilon > 0$ and $T > 0$,*

$$\mathbf{P}\left(\sup_{0 \leq t \leq T} |N(t) - t| \geq \epsilon \right) \leq 2e^{-Th(\epsilon/T)} ,$$

where $h(t) = (1 + t) \log(1 + t) - t$.

To prove this result, we rely on a classical result of martingale theory. Recall that a real-valued process $\{X(t)\}_{t \geq 0}$ is a martingale if and only if it satisfies

$$\mathbf{E}(X(t) \mid \{X(u)\}_{u \leq s}) = X(s), \ 0 \leq s \leq t.$$

If in this expression, the equality sign is replaced by the "greater than or equal to" sign, the process is a submartingale. We then have (see Williams [84]) the following:

Proposition 5.3 (Doob's inequality)   *Let $(X(t))_{t \geq 0}$ be a càdlàg (i.e. right-continuous with left limits) submartingale. Then for every $x \geq 0$ and $T \geq 0$, one has*

$$\mathbf{P}\left(\sup_{0 \leq t \leq T} |X(t)| \geq x \right) \leq \frac{1}{x} \mathbf{E}(|X(T)|) . \tag{5.1}$$

Proof of Proposition 5.2   Let $\theta > 0$ be fixed. By the union bound (also called Boole's inequality) and the fact that the exponential is an increasing function, we have

$$\mathbf{P}\left(\sup_{0 \leq t \leq T} |N(t) - t| \geq \epsilon \right)$$

$$\leq \mathbf{P}\left(\sup_{0 \leq t \leq T} (N(t) - t) \geq \epsilon \right) + \mathbf{P}\left(\sup_{0 \leq t \leq T} (t - N(t)) \geq \epsilon \right)$$

$$= \mathbf{P}\left(\sup_{0 \leq t \leq T} e^{\theta(N(t)-t)} \geq e^{\theta\epsilon} \right) + \mathbf{P}\left(\sup_{0 \leq t \leq T} e^{\theta(t-N(t))} \geq e^{\theta\epsilon} \right) .$$

Noting that both $(N(t) - t)_{t \geq 0}$ and $(t - N(t))_{t \geq 0}$ are martingales, we have by Jensen's inequality that the processes $(e^{\theta(N(t)-t)})_{t \geq 0}$ and $(e^{\theta(t-N(t))})_{t \geq 0}$ are non-negative submartingales. Therefore, by applying Doob's inequality, we obtain

$$\mathbf{P}\left(\sup_{0 \leq t \leq T} e^{\theta(N(t)-t)} \geq e^{\theta\epsilon} \right) \leq e^{-\theta\epsilon} \mathbf{E}\left(e^{\theta(N(T)-T)} \right) ,$$

$$\mathbf{P}\left(\sup_{0 \leq t \leq T} e^{-\theta(N(t)-t)} \geq e^{\theta\epsilon} \right) \leq e^{-\theta\epsilon} \mathbf{E}\left(e^{-\theta(N(T)-T)} \right) . \tag{5.2}$$

Using the fact that $N(T)$ is a Poisson random variable with parameter T, we obtain

$$\mathbf{P}\left(e^{\theta(N(t)-t)} \geq e^{\theta\epsilon} \right) \ \leq \ e^{-\theta(\epsilon+T)} \mathbf{E}\left(e^{\theta N(T)} \right)$$
$$= \ e^{-\theta(\epsilon+T)} e^{T(e^\theta - 1)}$$
$$= \ \exp\left(-\theta(\epsilon + T) + T(e^\theta - 1) \right) .$$

The exponent $-\theta(\epsilon+T)+T(e^\theta-1)$ can be minimised over the positive parameter θ by setting $\theta = \log(1 + \epsilon/T)$ (this is again an application of the Chernoff bounding technique). This yields

$$\mathbf{P}\left(\sup_{0 \leq t \leq T} (N(t) - t) \geq \epsilon \right) \leq e^{-Th(\epsilon/T)} ,$$

where $h(t) = (1 + t) \log (1 + t) - t$. Similarly, one obtains

$$\mathbf{P}\left(\sup_{0 \leq t \leq T} (t - N(t)) \geq \epsilon \right) \leq e^{-Th(-\epsilon/T)} .$$

The announced result follows from these bounds and the fact that $h(-x) \geq h(x)$, for $x \in [0, 1]$. $\qquad\qquad\square$

Example 5.4 **SIS epidemics.** The SIS (susceptible-infected-susceptible) process is defined as follows. There is a population of n individuals. Each individual can be either susceptible (S) or infected (I). Infected individuals infect someone else at rate β. They encounter other individuals uniformly at random from the whole population. If the target was susceptible, it becomes infected; if on the other hand it was already infected, nothing happens. In addition, each infected individual returns to the susceptible state at some rate δ.

Denote by $X_n(t)$ the number of infectives at time t. Then $\{X_n(t)\}_{t \geq 0}$ is an $\mathbb{N}$-valued birth and death process, with non-zero transition rates $\beta i(1 - i/n)$ from state i to state $i + 1$, and δi from state i to state $i - 1$. This in turn implies

$$
\begin{aligned}
\mathbf{P}(X_n(t + h) = i + 1 \mid X_n(t) = i) &= h \tfrac{\beta}{n} i(n - i) + o(h) , \\
\mathbf{P}(X_n(t + h) = i - 1 \mid X_n(t) = i) &= \delta i h + o(h) , \\
\mathbf{P}(X_n(t + h) = i \mid X_n(t) = i) &= 1 - h\left(\tfrac{\beta}{n} i(n - i) + \delta i \right) + o(h) .
\end{aligned}
$$

The result to follow will establish convergence, as n goes to infinity, of the trajectories $t \to \frac{1}{n} X_n(t)$ to the solution $x(t)$ of a simple differential equation.

5.3 Kurtz's theorem

Let the jump directions $(e_i)_{i=1,\dots,k}$, which are vectors in $\mathbb{Z}^d$, be given, together with corresponding functions $\lambda_i : \mathbb{R}^d \to \mathbb{R}_+$, $i \in \{1, \dots, k\}$. While for most examples of interest, the entries of these jump directions do belong to $\{-1, 0, 1\}$, we do not need to make this assumption in what follows.

For any $n \in \mathbb{N}$, we consider the Markov jump process $(X_n(t))_{t \in \mathbb{R}_+}$ on $\mathbb{N}^d$ with jump directions $(e_i)_{i=1,\dots,k}$ and corresponding transition rates $n\lambda_i(x/n)$, $x \in \mathbb{N}^d$ for the transition from $x \in \mathbb{N}^d$ to $x + e_i$. Thus the process $\{X_n(t)\}_{t \geq 0}$ satisfies

$$
\begin{aligned}
\mathbf{P}(X_n(t + h) = x + e_i \mid X_n(t) = x) &= nh\lambda_i(x/n) + o(h), \; x \in \mathbb{N}^d, \; i = 1, \dots, k, \\
\mathbf{P}(X_n(t + h) = x \mid X_n(t) = x) &= 1 - nh \textstyle\sum_{i=1}^{k} \lambda_i(x/n) + o(h) , \; x \in \mathbb{N}^d.
\end{aligned}
$$

Let the function $F : \mathbb{R}^d \to \mathbb{R}^d$ be defined by

$$F(x) := \sum_{i=1}^{k} e_i \lambda_i(x). \tag{5.3}$$

We then have the following result.

Theorem 5.5 (Kurtz's theorem)   *Let $\bar{e} := \max_{i=1,\ldots,k} |e_i|$ for some arbitrary norm $|\cdot|$. Assume that the supremum*

$$\bar{\lambda} := \max_{i=1,\ldots,k} \sup_{x\in\mathbb{R}^d} \lambda_i(x)$$

is finite, and that the function F defined by (5.3) is Lipschitz-continuous, i.e. there exists a constant M such that

$$|F(x) - F(y)| \le M|x - y|, \quad \text{for all } x, y \in \mathbb{R}^d.$$

Assume that $\lim_{n\to\infty} \frac{1}{n} X_n(0) = x(0)$, a.s., and let $x : \mathbb{R}_+ \to \mathbb{R}^d$ be the solution to the integral equation

$$x(t) = x(0) + \int_0^t F(x(s)) \, ds. \tag{5.4}$$

Then for any fixed $\epsilon, T > 0$, for sufficiently large n,

$$\mathbf{P}\left(\sup_{0\le t\le T} \left|\frac{1}{n} X_n(t) - x(t)\right| \ge \epsilon\right) \le 2k \exp\left(-nT\bar{\lambda}h\left(\frac{\epsilon e^{-MT}}{2kT\bar{\lambda}\bar{e}}\right)\right),$$

where $h(t) = (1 + t)\log(1 + t) - t$. Moreover,

$$\lim_{n\to\infty} \sup_{0\le t\le T} \left|\frac{1}{n} X_n(t) - x(t)\right| = 0, \quad a.s. \tag{5.5}$$

This theorem provides a law of large numbers for a sequence of birth and death processes as the size parameter n becomes large. Moreover, it provides a characterisation of the limiting process as the solution of a system of differential equations. Before we turn to its proof, let us illustrate its application on the SIS model.

For the SIS model, the two jump directions are $e_1 = +1$ and $e_2 = -1$, and the rate functions are $\lambda_1(x) = \beta x(1 - x)$, and $\lambda_2(x) = \gamma x$. Thus the function F reads

$$F(x) = \beta x(1 - x) - \delta x.$$

Assume without loss of generality (scaling time by some factor $\gamma = \delta^{-1}$) that $\delta = 1$. One can check that, for $\beta \ne 1$, the solution to the differential equation

$$\frac{dx}{dt} = F(x) = \beta x(1 - x) - x, \quad x(0) = y$$

is given by

$$x(t) = \frac{(\beta - 1)y e^{(\beta-1)t}}{(\beta - 1) - \beta y(1 - e^{(\beta-1)t})}. \tag{5.6}$$

Therefore, if $\beta > 1$, then $x(t) \to (1 - \frac{1}{\beta})$ as $t \to \infty$, whereas if $\beta < 1$, then $x(t) \to 0$ as $t \to \infty$.

Kurtz's theorem then implies that, for finite but large n, the state $X_n(t)$ is close to $nx(t)$, where $x(t)$ is given by Expression 5.6, and the initial condition $X_n(0)$ is given by ny.

Proof of Kurtz's theorem Let $(N_i)_{i=1,\dots,k}$ be independent unit-rate Poisson processes. Then we can construct the process $(X_n(t))_{t \in \mathbb{R}_+}$ as follows:

$$X_n(t) = X_n(0) + \sum_{i=1}^{k} e_i \, N_i \left(\int_0^t n\lambda_i \, (X(s)/n) \, ds \right).$$

Indeed, if $X(t) = x$, then there will be a jump in $N_i \left(\int_0^t n\lambda_i \, (X(s)/n) \, ds \right)$, during $(t, t+h)$ with probability $nh\lambda_i(x/n) + o(h)$, which corresponds to the probability of $X(t)$ having a jump in the direction e_i between t and $t + h$.

Introduce the notation $Y_n(t) = \frac{1}{n}X_n(t)$. The previous expression can then be rewritten as

$$Y_n(t) = Y_n(0) + \sum_{i=1}^{k} \frac{e_i}{n} \, \overline{N}_i \left(n \int_0^t \lambda_i \, (Y_n(s)) \, ds \right) + \int_0^t F(Y_n(s)) \, ds, \qquad (5.7)$$

where $\overline{N}_i(u) := N_i(u) - u$ is the centred Poisson process.

Subtracting (5.4), this implies that

$$\left| Y_n(t) - x(t) \right| \le \left| Y_n(0) - x(0) \right| + \int_0^t \left| F(Y_n(s)) - F(x(s)) \right| ds$$

$$+ \sum_{i=1}^{k} \frac{|e_i|}{n} \left| \overline{N}_i \left(n \int_0^t \lambda_i \, (X_n(s)) \, ds \right) \right|.$$

Using the fact that $\lim_{n \to \infty} Y_n(0) = x(0)$, a.s. and that F is M-Lipschitz, we have, for large n,

$$\left| Y_n(t) - x(t) \right| \le \epsilon + M \int_0^t \left| Y_n(s) - x(s) \right| ds + \sum_{i=1}^{k} \frac{1}{n} \epsilon_{n,i}(t), \qquad (5.8)$$

where $\epsilon_{n,i}(t) := |e_i| \cdot \left| \overline{N}_i \left(n \int_0^t \lambda_i \, (X_n(s)) \, ds \right) \right|$.

Applying Proposition 5.2, we obtain the following bound:

$$\mathbf{P}\left(\sup_{0\leq t\leq T}\sum_{i=1}^{k}\frac{1}{n}\epsilon_{n,i}(t)\geq \epsilon\right)\leq \sum_{i=1}^{k}\mathbf{P}\left(\sup_{0\leq t\leq T}\epsilon_{n,i}(t)\geq \frac{n\epsilon}{k}\right)$$

$$\leq \sum_{i=1}^{k}\mathbf{P}\left(\sup_{0\leq t\leq nT\bar{\lambda}}\bar{e}\left|\overline{N}(t)\right|\geq \frac{n\epsilon}{k}\right)$$

$$\leq 2ke^{-nT\bar{\lambda}h\left(\frac{\epsilon}{kT\bar{\lambda}\bar{e}}\right)}. \tag{5.9}$$

Combining (5.8) and (5.9) yields:

$$\mathbf{P}\left(\sup_{0\leq t\leq T}\left[\left|Y_n(t)-x(t)\right|-M\int_0^t\left|Y_n(s)-x(s)\right|ds\right]\geq 2\epsilon\right)$$

$$\leq 2k\exp\left(-nT\bar{\lambda}h\left(\frac{\epsilon}{kT\bar{\lambda}\bar{e}}\right)\right). \tag{5.10}$$

We now need the following result.

Proposition 5.6 (Gronwall's lemma)   *Let u be a bounded real-valued function on $[0,T]$ satisfying*

$$u(t)\leq a+b\int_0^t u(s)\,ds, \quad \text{for all } t\in[0,T], \tag{5.11}$$

where a and b are non-zero constants. Then

$$u(t)\leq ae^{bt}.$$

Proof   Let $v(t)=e^{-bt}\int_0^t u(s)\,ds$. Then

$$\begin{aligned}
v'(t) &= -be^{-bt}\int_0^t u(s)\,ds+e^{-bt}u(t)\\
&\leq -be^{-bt}\int_0^t u(s)\,ds+ae^{-bt}+be^{-bt}\int_0^t u(s)\,ds\\
&= ae^{-bt}.
\end{aligned}$$

Integrating from 0 to t, we obtain

$$v(t)\leq \frac{a}{b}(1-e^{-bt}).$$

Replacing $v(t)$ by its full expression we obtain

$$\int_0^t u(s)\,ds\leq \frac{a}{b}(e^{bt}-1).$$

Hence, by (5.11)

$$u(t)\leq a+b\int_0^t u(s)\,ds\leq a+a(e^{bt}-1)=ae^{bt}.$$

$\square$

It is not difficult to check that the function $|Y_n(t) - x(t)|$ is bounded, with probability 1, on the interval $[0, T]$. Let $Z_n(t) = |Y_n(t) - x(t)|$ for n an integer and t a non-negative real. Applying Gronwall's lemma to the function $|Y_n(t) - x(t)|$ yields

$$\mathbf{P}\left(\sup_{0 \leq t \leq T} |Y_n(t) - x(t)| \geq 2\epsilon e^{MT} \right)$$
$$\leq \mathbf{P}\left(\sup_{0 \leq t \leq T} \left[Z_n(t) - M \int_0^t Z_n(s)ds \right] \geq 2\epsilon \right)$$
$$\leq 2k e^{-nT\bar{\lambda}h\left(\frac{\epsilon}{kT\bar{\lambda}\bar{e}} \right)},$$

or alternatively,

$$\mathbf{P}\left(\sup_{0 \leq t \leq T} |Y_n(t) - x(t)| \geq \epsilon \right) \leq 2k e^{-nT\bar{\lambda}h\left(\frac{\epsilon e^{-MT}}{2kT\bar{\lambda}\bar{e}} \right)}.$$

Hence $\sum_{n \in \mathbb{N}} \mathbf{P}\left(\sup_{0 \leq t \leq T} |Y_n(t) - x(t)| \geq \epsilon \right) < \infty$, and the almost sure convergence in (5.5) follows immediately by the Borel–Cantelli lemma. $\square$

5.4 Notes

A more general derivation of Kurtz's theorem is described in Ethier and Kurtz [32], together with diffusion approximations. In Andersson and Britton [3], differential equation approximations of classical epidemic models are derived using a weaker version of Kurtz's theorem. A detailed analysis of several deterministic approximations of epidemics and rumour models is given in Daley and Gani [23]. Kurtz's theorem is an important tool in analysing many problems related to networks, such as peer-to-peer systems (Massoulié and Vojovnic [64]), reputation systems in social networks (Mundinger and Le Boudec [73]) and communication protocols (e.g. Ganesh *et al.* [37] and Kumar and Massoulié [50]).

PART II

STRUCTURED NETWORKS

6

The small-world phenomenon

6.1 Introduction

In 1967, the sociologist Stanley Milgram published [65] results of a letter-relaying experiment of his design. The now-famous experiment required a source individual to forward a letter to a destination individual, about whom was disclosed information such as address, name and profession. However, each source individual was forbidden to post the letter directly to the target person. Instead she was required to forward the letter to someone known on a first-name basis, who in turn was allowed to forward it only to such familiar contacts.

The outcome was that a significant fraction of letters reached their destinations. Moreover, they did so in at most six hops, justifying the term "six degrees of separation". This observation is also often referred to as the "small-world phenomenon". The problem, formulated in the social sciences, is highly relevant in many other settings, namely routing with limited information in communication networks and browsing behaviour on the World Wide Web.

Viewing the social world as a graph with edges between acquainted persons, if any individual can relay information to any other in a small number of hops as in Milgram's experiment, the corresponding graph must have a small diameter. As we saw in Chapter 4, the E-R graph does have a small diameter (logarithmic in the number of nodes). However, this graph is not a realistic model of social graphs, because it possesses no structure, whereas social graphs are affected by geographic location of individuals and area of professional activity among many factors.

If in Milgram's experiment one were allowed to "spam" one's acquaintances with duplicates of the letter, then the outcome could be seen as the unfolding of an epidemic, or the spreading of a rumour, on a social network. We are thus interested in identifying network structures which allow for fast propagation, and yet display structure as social networks do. We are also interested in identifying schemes that leverage such structure to enable fast propagation of information.

In this chapter we discuss two models to explain how such structures arise. We first examine a variant of some of the models studied by physicists Strogatz and Watts (see e.g. [82]) to illustrate how graphs with spatial structure can also exhibit small diameters, hence providing more realistic models of social graphs. We then explore an algorithmic setting that highlights the small-world phenomenon.

6.2 Small world according to Strogatz and Watts

Given some integer $m > 0$, the node set of the graph is the set of points $(i, j) \in \{1, \ldots, m\} \times \{1, \ldots, m\}$ in two-dimensional Cartesian space. There are thus $n = m^2$ nodes. These nodes are connected via two types of edges: local edges to grid neighbours (see Figure 6.1, *left*), and thus between 2 and 4 such edges per node (accounting for boundary effects), and "shortcut" edges. The latter are generated as follows.

The model features a second parameter, $p \in (0, 1)$. Each node u, with probability p, creates a shortcut edge, whose other endpoint is chosen uniformly at random from the node set. We denote by $SW(n, p)$ the corresponding random graph.

Note that without the addition of shortcuts, the diameter of the graph would be $2m = 2\sqrt{n}$. We now show that for any fixed $p > 0$, the presence of shortcuts will radically reduce the graph's diameter.

Theorem 6.1 *Let $p > 0$ be fixed. Then for some constant A depending on p, the diameter $D(SW)$ of the graph SW, satisfies*

$$\lim_{n \to \infty} \mathbf{P}(D(SW(n, p)) \leq A \log(n)) = 1 .$$

The proof will proceed by reducing the graph $SW(n, p)$ to a graph G' whose nodes are clusters of the nodes of $SW(n, p)$ of size k as illustrated in Figure 6.1 (the squares on the right correspond to clusters of nodes from the graph on the left, and the links between these clusters are inherited from the original graph as described below). This construction will enable us to find an upper bound on the diameter of $SW(n, p)$ in terms of the diameter of G'. To bound the diameter of G' we derive a result that is analogous to Lemma 4.4 in the context of E-R graphs. The proof is however more intricate as it requires the use of the Azuma–Hoeffding inequality, to be introduced shortly.

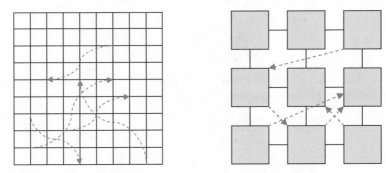

Figure 6.1 Strogatz–Watts graph and induced graph G'

Proof For some integer k such that $kp > 1$, cut the grid into squares of k nodes (we choose k so that $\sqrt{k}$ is an integer and assume it divides m; this restriction loses no generality). We shall work on the graph G' whose nodes correspond to these squares; neighbouring squares are connected by local edges; each square generates a random number of shortcut edges, whose distribution is now binomial with parameters (k, p). The other endpoints of these shortcuts are drawn uniformly from the node set of G'. We shall denote by $\mathcal{N}'$ the node set of G', and let $n' = n/k$ be the number of nodes.

Note that the diameters of SW and G' satisfy

$$D(SW) \leq 2\sqrt{k}\,(2 + D(G'))\,.$$

Indeed, given two nodes u', v' of SW, let u, v denote the corresponding nodes in G'. Given a path in G' of length not larger than $D(G')$, one can construct from it a path in SW of not more than $2\sqrt{k}\,(D(G') + 2)$ hops, hence the result. From now on we aim to bound the diameter of G'.

Let $\Gamma_1(u)$ denote a group of nodes containing u, of size $C \log n$ for some suitable constant C, and such that the nodes of $\Gamma_1(u)$ are all connected via grid edges. We shall denote by $\Gamma_2(u)$ the nodes reached from nodes in $\Gamma_1(u)$ via shortcuts generated from $\Gamma_1(u)$, and similarly we define $\Gamma_i(u)$ for $i > 2$ as the sets of new nodes reached by shortcuts created in $\Gamma_{i-1}(u)$. As in the study of the E-R graph, for nodes $u \in \mathcal{N}'$ of G', and $i \geq 0$, we use the notation $d_i(u) = |\Gamma_i(u)|$. The following result is the counterpart of Lemma 4.4 in the present context.

Lemma 6.2 *Let $\epsilon > 0$ be fixed, such that*

$$kp(1 - \epsilon) > 1\,, \tag{6.1}$$

and

$$\frac{\log(kp(1 + \epsilon))}{\log(kp(1 - \epsilon))} < 2 \,. \tag{6.2}$$

The constant $C > 0$ can be chosen so that, for all $u \in N'$, with probability $1 - o(n^{-2})$, the following inequalities hold:

$$kp(1 - \epsilon) \leq \frac{d_i(u)}{d_{i-1}(u)} \leq kp(1 + \epsilon), \quad i = 2, \ldots, D, \tag{6.3}$$

where $D = \lceil \log(n)/2 \log(kp(1 - \epsilon)) \rceil + 1$.

Before giving the proof of the lemma, we state the so-called the Azuma–Hoeffding inequality [67], which will play the role of the Chernoff bound, since we need to deal with correlated indicator variables rather than independent ones.

Theorem 6.3 (Azuma–Hoeffding inequality)   *Let $\{M_t\}_{t=0,\ldots,T}$ be a martingale such that for all $t = 1, \ldots, T$,*

$$|M_t - M_{t-1}| \leq c_t \text{ almost surely} \tag{6.4}$$

for positive constants $c_1, \ldots, c_T$. Then for all $x > 0$, one has

$$\mathbf{P}(M_T - M_0 \geq x) \leq \exp\left(-\frac{x^2}{2 \sum_{t=1}^{T} c_t^2}\right). \tag{6.5}$$

Proof   Fix $\theta > 0$. Chebyshev's inequality yields

$$\mathbf{P}(M_T - M_0 \geq x) \leq \mathbf{E}\left[\exp(\theta(M_{T-1} - M_0))\mathbf{E}\left(\exp(\theta(M_T - M_{T-1})) \mid \mathcal{F}_{T-1}\right)\right] e^{-\theta x}, \tag{6.6}$$

where $\mathcal{F}_t = \sigma(M_0, \ldots, M_t)$, the sigma algebra generated by $M_0, \ldots, M_t$. Note that, in view of assumption (6.4), for some $Z \in [0, 1]$, one has

$$M_T - M_{T-1} = Zc_T + (1 - Z)(-c_T) \,.$$

Thus by convexity of the function $y \to e^{\theta y}$, one has

$$\exp(\theta(M_T - M_{T-1})) \leq Ze^{\theta c_T} + (1 - Z)e^{-\theta c_T} \,.$$

Furthermore, by the martingale property, $\mathbf{E}(M_T - M_{T-1} \mid \mathcal{F}_{T-1}) = 0$. Equivalently, $\mathbf{E}(Z \mid \mathcal{F}_{T-1}) = 1/2$, so that

$$\mathbf{E}(\exp(\theta(M_T - M_{T-1})) \mid \mathcal{F}_{T-1}) \leq \frac{e^{\theta c_T} + e^{-\theta c_T}}{2} \,.$$

Expanding the right-hand side in power series of θc_T, it can be seen that this is less than or equal to $\exp((\theta c_T)^2/2)$. Repeating the argument, we obtain from (6.6)

$$P(M_T - M_0 \geq x) \leq \exp\left(\frac{\theta^2 \sum_{t=1}^{T} c_t^2}{2}\right)\exp(-\theta x).$$

Optimising over $\theta > 0$ yields the result (6.5). □

The theorem has a useful corollary.

Corollary 6.4 *Let $f : \Omega_1 \times \cdots \times \Omega_T \to \mathbb{R}$ be a measurable function such that, for all $x_1, \ldots, x_T \in \Omega_1 \times \cdots \times \Omega_T$, all $t \in \{1, \ldots, T\}$ and all $y_t \in \Omega_t$, one has*

$$|f(x) - f(x_1, \ldots, x_{t-1}, y_t, x_{t+1}, \ldots, x_T)| \leq c_t. \tag{6.7}$$

Then, given independent random variables $X_1, \ldots, X_T$ taking their values in $\Omega_1, \ldots, \Omega_T$ respectively, the random variable $Y := f(X_1, \ldots, X_T)$ satisfies for all $x > 0$

$$P(Y - E(Y) \geq x) \leq \exp\left(-\frac{x^2}{2\sum_{t=1}^{T} c_t^2}\right).$$

Proof For all $t = 0, \ldots T$, let $M_t = E(Y \mid X_1, \ldots, X_t)$; in particular, $M_0 = E(Y)$ and $M_T = Y$. Let us verify that the martingale $\{M_t\}_{0 \leq t \leq T}$ satisfies assumption (6.4). Let $p_t(\cdot)$ denote the probability distribution of X_t. For all $t = 1, \ldots, T$, one has

$$|M_t - M_{t-1}| = \left|\int_{\Omega_t \times \cdots \times \Omega_T} p_t(dy_t) \times \cdots \times p_T(dy_T)\left[f\left(X_1^t y_{t+1}^T\right) - f\left(X_1^{t-1} y_t^T\right)\right]\right|$$
$$\leq c_t$$

in view of assumption (6.7), where we use the notation

$$\left(x_1^t y_{t+1}^T\right) = (x_1, \ldots, x_t, y_{t+1}, \ldots, y_T).$$

The result follows. □

Returning to the proof of Lemma 6.2, note that conditional on $d_1(u), \ldots, d_{i-1}(u)$ the number of shortcuts generated from $\Gamma_{i-1}(u)$ follows a binomial distribution with parameters $(kd_{i-1}(u), p)$. Let T denote this number of shortcuts.

Condition on the number T and on the sets $\Gamma_1(u), \ldots, \Gamma_{i-1}(u)$, and let the nodes to which these shortcuts connect be denoted by $A_1, \ldots, A_T$. Writing $d_i(u) = f(A_1, \ldots, A_T)$, it is readily seen that function f satisfies condition (6.7) of Corollary 6.4 with $c_t = 1$. Indeed, we can view $d_i(u)$ as counting the number of occupied bins, among the $n' - 1 - d_1(u) - \ldots - d_{i-1}(u)$ bins available, after throwing T balls at random. Changing the location of one ball can change the number of occupied bins by at most 1. We thus have

$$\mathbf{P}\left(d_i(u) - \bar{d}_i(u) \geq x \mid T, \Gamma_1(u), \ldots, \Gamma_{i-1}(u)\right) \leq \exp\left(-\frac{x^2}{2T}\right),$$

where $\bar{d}_i(u) = \mathbf{E}\left(d_i(u) \mid T, \Gamma_1(u), \ldots, \Gamma_{i-1}(u)\right)$. The same upper bound holds for deviations of $d_i(u) - \bar{d}_i(u)$ below $-x$, by symmetry. Note that

$$\bar{d}_i(u) = (n' - 1 - d_1(u) - \cdots - d_{i-1}(u))(1 - (1 - 1/n')^T).$$

Denote by $\mathcal{E}_i(u)$ the event

$$\mathcal{E}_i(u) = \{(1 - \epsilon)kp \leq d_i(u)/d_{i-1}(u) \leq (1 + \epsilon)kp\}.$$

Let $\mathcal{I} := [kpd_{i-1}(u)(1 - \epsilon/2), kpd_{i-1}(u)(1 + \epsilon/2)]$. Letting $\bar{\mathcal{E}}_i(u)$ be the complement of $\mathcal{E}_i(u)$, we have

$$\mathbf{P}\left(\bar{\mathcal{E}}_i(u) \mid \mathcal{E}_2(u), \ldots, \mathcal{E}_{i-1}(u)\right)$$

$$\leq \mathbf{P}(T \notin \mathcal{I} \mid \mathcal{E}_2(u), \ldots, \mathcal{E}_{i-1}(u))$$

$$+ \mathbf{P}\left(\frac{d_i(u)}{d_{i-1}(u)} \geq kp(1 + \epsilon) \mid T \in \mathcal{I}, \mathcal{E}_2(u), \ldots, \mathcal{E}_{i-1}(u)\right) \qquad (6.8)$$

$$+ \mathbf{P}\left(\frac{d_i(u)}{d_{i-1}(u)} \leq kp(1 - \epsilon) \mid T \in \mathcal{I}, \mathcal{E}_2(u), \ldots, \mathcal{E}_{i-1}(u)\right).$$

Conditional on the event $\bigcap_{j=2}^{i-1} \mathcal{E}_j(u)$, since $kp(1 - \epsilon) > 1$ by assumption (6.1), and that $d_1(u) = C\log(n)$ by construction, it holds that

$$d_{i-1}(u) \geq C\log n.$$

Thus, using lemma 2.4, the first term on the right-hand side of inequality (6.8) is bounded by $2\exp\left(-(C\log n)h(\epsilon/2)\right)$. For suitably large C, this is less than n^{-K} for any desired $K > 0$.

The Azuma–Hoeffding inequality yields the following bound on the second term on the right-hand side of (6.8):

$$\sup_{T \in \mathcal{I}} \exp\left(-x^2/(2T)\right),$$

where

$$x = d_{i-1}(u)kp(1 + \epsilon) - (n' - 1 - d_1(u) - \cdots - d_{i-1}(u))(1 - (1 - 1/n')^T).$$

Using condition (6.2), it can be shown that for all $i \leq D$, conditional on the event $\bigcap_{j=2}^{i-1} \mathcal{E}_j(u)$, one has $d_{i-1}(u) = o(n)$. It follows that x in the expression above is bounded below by $d_{i-1}(u)kp(1 + \epsilon) - (1 + o(1))T$, and eventually the Azuma–Hoeffding bound is bounded above by $\exp(-\epsilon'(C\log n))$ for some suitable $\epsilon' > 0$. The third term on the right-hand side of (6.8) is dealt with in a similar manner. Eventually, we obtain that for any $K > 0$, and for a suitable choice of C, for all u and all $i = 1, \ldots, D$,

$$\mathbf{P}\left(\bar{\mathcal{E}}_i \mid \mathcal{E}_2(u), \ldots, \mathcal{E}_{i-1}(u)\right) \leq n^{-K}.$$

The result of Lemma 6.2 readily follows.

The proof of Theorem 6.1 is now concluded as follows. Given any two nodes u, v, we have

$$\mathbf{P}(d_{G'}(u, v) > 2D + 2C \log(n)) \leq \mathbf{P}\left(\overline{\bigcap_{i=2}^{D} \mathcal{E}_i(u)}\right) + \mathbf{P}\left(\overline{\bigcap_{i=2}^{D} \mathcal{E}_i(v)}\right) + \pi,$$

where π is the probability that two sets of sizes $(C \log n)kp(1 - \epsilon)^D$, picked uniformly at random from a set of n nodes, have an empty intersection. Note that

$$(C \log n)kp(1 - \epsilon)^D \geq r = (C \log n) \sqrt{n},$$

by our choice of D. In view of Lemma 4.5, we thus have that

$$\pi \leq (1 + o(1)) \exp\left(-C^2(\log n)^2(1 + o(1))\right).$$

Thus certainly, $\mathbf{P}(d_{G'}(u, v) > 2D + 2C \log n) = o(n^{-2})$. Summing this evaluation over all pairs (u, v) ensures that with high probability, the diameter of G' is $O(\log n)$. □

6.3 Small world according to Kleinberg

In 2000, Kleinberg [46] revisited the small-world phenomenon. His key observation is that while models such as the Strogatz–Watts graph can explain the presence of short paths between nodes, they do not explain how individuals managed to efficiently determine such short paths in Milgram's experiment.

Indeed, the original Milgram experiment contains a striking algorithmic aspect: not only do short paths exist in the social network, but individuals were collectively able to find short paths to their targets using only limited personal knowledge at each step. In some sense the network contained structure that each individual could leverage to have their letter reach its target in only a few hops. This property, sometimes called navigability, is not captured in our analysis of the Strogatz and Watts model.

Kleinberg proposes a model related to that of Strogatz and Watts, but where the distribution of the destination of shortcuts is not necessarily uniform. A parameter α characterises this distribution of shortcuts. Kleinberg showed that, for a critical value α^* of α, individuals can determine paths of length at most a power of the logarithm of the number of nodes. He also established that, for $\alpha < \alpha^*$, short paths exist but individuals cannot determine them in a decentralised manner, i.e. based on the mere knowledge of the underlying grid structure, the location of the target, and individual long-range contacts. When $\alpha > \alpha^*$, short paths no longer exist. As a result, unless $\alpha = \alpha^*$, in this model it takes a number of steps that is on the order of a power of the number of nodes, instead of its logarithm, for an individual to reach another specified individual.

6.3.1 The model

As for the Strogatz–Watts model, nodes are identified with the points of the grid $\{1, \ldots, m\} \times \{1, \ldots, m\}$. Nodes u and v are grid neighbours if their L^1 distance $|u - v| = |u_1 - v_1| + |u_2 - v_2|$ equals 1. An additional parameter q determines the number of shortcuts generated by each individual. Finally, a node u chooses another node v as the destination of a shortcut with probability $|u - v|^{-\alpha} / \sum_{w \neq u} |u - w|^{-\alpha}$, for some parameter $\alpha \geq 0$. Here, $|u - v|$ refers to the minimal number of hops from u to v using grid edges only, or equivalently the L^1 distance.

Note that when $\alpha = 0$, shortcuts are again selected uniformly at random (the case $\alpha = 0, q = 1$ corresponds to the Strogatz–Watts graph described in Section 6.2). Thus, by the analysis of the model of Strogatz and Watts, we know that, in this case, the diameter is logarithmic in the number of nodes $n = m^2$.

6.3.2 Efficient routing for critical α

In this section we show that efficient routing can be performed when $\alpha = 2$. To this end we will describe a greedy decentralised (or distributed) scheme that consists of always forwarding the message to a grid node as close as possible to the target.[1]

Theorem 6.5 *Assume $\alpha = 2$. Consider the following greedy routing scheme. A node u, trying to reach a node v, forwards the message to the node w among its grid and shortcut neighbours that is closest (according to L^1 distance) to the target v. Then, for all nodes u, v, the number of steps $T_{greedy}(u, v)$ used by this scheme to reach v from u satisfies*

$$\mathbf{E}(T_{greedy}(u, v)) \leq O(\log n)^2 . \tag{6.9}$$

---

[1] A *greedy* algorithm is an algorithm that always makes the choice that looks best at each moment.

Proof   Let the source and destination nodes u, v be fixed. Let $u(t)$ be the node to which the greedy algorithm has forwarded the message after t steps. We shall say that the algorithm is "in phase j" at time t if

$$2^j < |u(t) - v| \le 2^{j+1} .$$

At each step spent in phase j, at least one new shortcut is discovered (recall that $q \ge 1$ shortcuts are created from each node; also, the presence of grid edges guarantees that the greedy algorithm moves closer to the destination at each step). Assuming $u(t)$ belongs to phase j, the probability that a shortcut to a node w leads to a phase $k < j$ admits the lower bound

$$\min_{u(t):2^j<|u(t)-v|\le 2^{j+1}} \frac{\sum_{w:|v-w|\le 2^j} |u(t) - w|^{-2}}{\sum_{u' \neq u(t)} |u(t) - u'|^{-2}} .$$

The numerator is always greater than

$$(2^{j+1} + 2^j)^{-2} \sum_{i=1}^{2^j} i \ge 1/36 ,$$

while the denominator is always less than

$$\sum_{i=1}^{2m} (4i) i^{-2} \le 4 \left(1 + \int_1^{2m} \frac{1}{x} \, dx \right) \le 4(1 + \log 2m) .$$

Thus the probability of moving to a better phase is at least

$$\frac{1}{144(1 + \log 2m)} .$$

So the number of steps spent in a given phase j is stochastically dominated by a geometric random variable with parameter $1/[144(1 + \log 2m)]$. Since there are at most $\log_2 2m$ phases, the average number of steps needed to reach the destination satisfies

$$\mathbf{E}\left(T_{greedy}(u, v)\right) \le 144(1 + \log 2m) \frac{\log 2m}{\log 2} = O((\log n)^2) ,$$

as claimed.   □

6.3.3 Impossibility of efficient routing, $\alpha < 2$

In the present context, we say that a routing algorithm is decentralised, or distributed, if the routing decision made at step t depends only on knowledge of the nodes $u(0), \ldots, u(t)$ visited so far, and on the knowledge of the coordinates of the destinations of shortcuts generated at these nodes. Clearly, the greedy algorithm used in Theorem 6.5 is decentralised in this sense.

We now show that for $\alpha < 2$, no decentralised algorithm can perform efficiently.

Theorem 6.6 *Assume $\alpha \in [0, 2)$. Then for any decentralised algorithm alg, the average number of steps $E\left[T_{alg}(u, v)\right]$ needed to reach a destination v from a source u satisfies, for "most" pairs (u, v),*

$$E\left[T_{alg}(u, v)\right] = \Omega\left(m^{(2-\alpha)/3}\right) . \tag{6.10}$$

In other words, there is a constant $\delta > 0$ such that

$$E\left[T_{alg}(u, v)\right] \geq \delta\left(m^{(2-\alpha)/3}\right) .$$

Proof Consider the neighbourhood $\mathcal{V} = \{w : |v - w| \leq C\}$, for some C to be specified, and let $t = \epsilon C$, for some fixed $\epsilon \in (0, 1)$. Assume that $|u - v| > C$. Then, if the algorithm is to reach v from u in t steps, the last shortcut used by the algorithm must end in neighbourhood $\mathcal{V}$. Otherwise, after the last shortcut is taken, the current node will be outside $\mathcal{V}$; however, there remain at most $t < C$ steps to take, and using only grid edges this will not reach v from outside $\mathcal{V}$, by definition of $\mathcal{V}$.

Thus the algorithm will fail to route to destination in t steps if it does not discover a shortcut leading into $\mathcal{V}$ in the first t visited locations. From any node w, the probability that a shortcut generated at that node reaches $\mathcal{V}$ is

$$\frac{\sum_{v':|v'-v|\leq C} |v' - w|^{-\alpha}}{\sum_{v'\neq w} |v' - w|^{-\alpha}} .$$

The numerator is bounded from above, uniformly in w, by $|\mathcal{V}|$, which is no larger than $1 + 4C(C + 1)/2$, itself not larger than $3C^2$ for $C \geq 1$. The denominator is bounded below by

$$\sum_{i=1}^{m/2} i \times i^{-\alpha} \geq \int_1^{m/2} x^{1-\alpha} dx = \frac{(m/2)^{2-\alpha} - 1}{2 - \alpha} \geq \frac{m^{2-\alpha}}{2^{3-\alpha}}$$

for m large enough. Thus the probability of a shortcut reaching $\mathcal{V}$ is at most $6C^2 m^{\alpha-2}$. Finally, since at each step at most q new shortcuts are discovered, by the argument above the probability of failing to route to destination in t steps is at least

$$1 - qt \sup_w P(\text{shortcut generated from } w \text{ reaches } \mathcal{V}) \geq 1 - q\epsilon\left(6C^3 m^{\alpha-2}/2^{3-\alpha}\right) .$$

Setting $C = \left(\frac{m^{(2-\alpha)}}{2^{3-\alpha}}\right)^{1/3}$ and $\epsilon = 1/(12q)$, the right-hand side simplifies to $1/2$. Finally, we obtain that, for u, v such that $|u - v| > m^{(2-\alpha)/3}$,

$$E\left[T_{alg}(u, v)\right] \geq \delta \cdot m^{(2-\alpha)/3}, \text{ for some constant } \delta > 0.$$

Since the fraction of pairs of nodes (u, v) such that $|u-v| > m^{(2-\alpha)/3}$ approaches 1 as $m \to \infty$, the claim follows. $\square$

6.3.4 Impossibility of efficient routing, $\alpha > 2$

In this section we prove that, if the parameter α is larger than 2, any distributed scheme will take a positive power of n steps to pass the message from any source to any destination.

Theorem 6.7 *Assume that $\alpha > 2$. There is an increasing function $f : \mathbb{R}^+ \to \mathbb{R}^+$ such that, for any distributed algorithm alg, and any source and destination nodes u, v, the expected number of steps from source to destination satisfies*

$$\mathbf{E}\left[T_{alg}(u, v)\right] \geq f\left(|u - v|/m\right) m^\gamma , \qquad (6.11)$$

where $\gamma := (\alpha - 2)/(\alpha - 1)$. Thus, for more than one half (say) of pairs of nodes u, v, decentralised routing takes on the order of m^γ steps on average.

Proof For some d (to be specified), note that the probability that a shortcut generated at a node w reaches a target w' such that $|w - w'|$ exceeds d is at most

$$\frac{\sum_{i=d+1}^{\infty} 4i \times i^{-\alpha}}{\sum_{w' \neq w} |w - w'|^{-\alpha}} \leq 4 \int_d^{\infty} x^{1-\alpha} dx = \frac{4}{2 - \alpha} d^{\alpha-2} .$$

Given a target number of steps t, and two nodes u, v, such that $td < |u - v|$, routing from source u will fail to reach destination v in t steps if shortcuts found in these t steps all have length not larger than d. This implies

$$\mathbf{E}\left[T_{alg}(u, v)\right] \geq t\left[1 - qt\frac{4}{\alpha - 2}d^{\alpha-2}\right] . \qquad (6.12)$$

Now choose t, d to ensure

$$td = \frac{|u - v|}{2} ,$$

and

$$qt\frac{4}{\alpha - 2}d^{2-\alpha} = 1/2 ,$$

the latter ensuring that the right-hand side in (6.12) equals $1/2$. Solving these two equations gives

$$d = |u - v|^{1/(\alpha-1)}\left[\frac{4q}{\alpha - 2}\right]^{1/(\alpha-1)} , \quad t = |u - v|^{(\alpha-2)/(\alpha-1)}\frac{1}{2}\left[\frac{4q}{\alpha - 2}\right]^{-1/(\alpha-1)} .$$

Evaluation (6.11) now follows from (6.12) by setting

$$f(x) = x^\gamma \frac{1}{4}\left[\frac{4q}{\alpha - 2}\right]^{-1/(\alpha-1)} . \qquad \square$$

6.4 Notes

A discussion by Kleinberg relating his perspective to that of Strogatz and Watts can be found in [47]. The seminal work of Kleinberg has led to numerous studies that attempt to achieve deeper understanding of small-world (aka navigable) networks.

First, a number of papers have studied the effect of providing small amounts of additional information to the message holder. For example, Labhar and Schabanel [53] consider algorithms where the message holder can consult a set of nearby nodes to get the best shortcut, yielding shorter routes.

Several recent papers consider navigable networks on underlying structures other than the grid; in particular, Draief and Ganesh [26] examine the continuous analogue of Kleinberg's model and show that similar results hold (see Franceschetti and Meester [35] for a discussion of continuous models in the context of communication networks). More recently, Duchon *et al.* [52] have examined whether any graph can be turned into a small-world graph by the addition of shortcuts. Finally, Lebhar, Chaintreau and Fraigniaud [51] describe a dynamic process on the grid whereby nodes create shortcuts by moving on the network and discovering other nodes. They show that in the "long run" this model yields shortcuts à la Kleinberg and therefore a navigable network.

7

Power laws via preferential attachment

7.1 Introduction

So far we have considered E-R random graphs, de Bruijn graphs and small-world graphs à la Strogatz and Watts or à la Kleinberg. In all these examples, the degree distribution of nodes is sharply concentrated around its mean. For E-R graphs on n nodes, using the Chernoff bound described in Chapter 2, Lemma 2.4, denoting by δ the average degree $\delta = (n-1)p$, it holds that, for d_i the degree (number of neighbours) of node i:

$$\mathbf{P}\left(\exists i \in \{1, \ldots, n\} : |d_i - \delta| \geq \epsilon\delta\right) \leq n\left(\exp(-\delta h(\epsilon)) + \exp(-\delta h(-\epsilon))\right).$$

Thus, assuming $\delta \gg \log n$, if we take $\epsilon = 2\sqrt{(\log n)/\delta}$, since $h(x) = (1 + o(x))x^2/2$, we find that the exponents on the right-hand side above are equivalent to $2\log n$, hence the right-hand side is of order $1/n$: with high probability, no node degree deviates from the mean degree δ by a factor larger than $2\sqrt{(\log n)/\delta} \ll 1$.

The degrees in all the other graphs we have studied so far are, with high probability, bounded by a constant multiple of the logarithm $\log n$ of the number of nodes n. By contrast, many examples of graphs display very different degree distributions. In particular, it is common to have graphs where the fraction of nodes of degree i is roughly proportional to $i^{-\beta}$, for some exponent $\beta > 2$, and over a significant range of values i. Networks with such degree distribution are known as *power-law graphs*.

In this chapter we present a model that yields power-law graphs with $\beta > 3$. We do not attempt to provide a rigorous definition, or to make precise what is meant by "roughly proportional" and "significant range of values". Examples where this behaviour appears are the graph of the Internet topology, when viewed at the router level and also at the autonomous system level; the web graph, in which nodes are web pages and links are hyperlinks; and the "Hollywood graph", where nodes are actors and links indicate that two actors appeared in the same movie. For a survey with many more examples, see Newman [76]. The power-law property of graphs also has implications for the behaviour of processes such as epidemics that may evolve on them.

Given the importance of the power-law property, as well as its ubiquity, it is of interest to understand its origin. This chapter is thus concerned with generative models that produce graphs with such properties. The benefit of generating such graphs is twofold. First, it illuminates how global properties of this sort arise from a set of local rules that dictate the way in which links are formed between nodes. Second, we can use these graphs as benchmarks for studying the behaviour of dynamic processes on such networks both analytically and through simulation.

One mechanism that has been proposed for explaining the presence of power laws is that of *preferential attachment*. We shall first illustrate this on a simple graph formation process, which has been popularised by Barabási and Albert [8]. We will then present a precursor of this model, namely the model of Yule [86] for explaining power-law distributions for the number of species within genera of plants (among other broad families of living things).

Another interesting feature of the analyses of both the Barabási–Albert and the Yule models is that they provide a very nice illustration of the use of the Azuma–Hoeffding inequality, justified by a coupling construction.

7.2 Barabási-Albert random graphs

We consider the following model. A graph is grown over time, starting with an initial graph $G(0)$, and adding one node $u(t)$ at each time step $t = 1, 2, \ldots$. The resulting graph at the end of step t is denoted $G(t)$ and has

$$N(t) = N(0) + t$$

nodes. The new node $u(t)$ is attached to the previous graph $G(t-1)$ by a single edge. Thus the total number of edges in $G(t)$, which we denote $E(t)$, satisfies

$$E(t) = E(0) + t.$$

The node to which $u(t + 1)$ attaches in $G(t)$ is chosen as follows. For some parameter $\alpha \in (0, 1)$, the anchor node is chosen uniformly at random from the $N(t)$ nodes of $G(t)$ with probability α. With probability $1 - \alpha$, a node v is selected with probability $d_t(v)/2E(t)$, where $d_t(v)$ denotes the degree of node v in graph $G(t)$. This defines a proper probability distribution because the sum of node degrees in $G(t)$ is indeed twice the number of edges $E(t)$. In other words, when a new node joins the system, it either randomly creates a link or it links to nodes that are already popular, i.e. have many neighbours. This construction is known as a preferential attachment scheme since nodes with a high degree (large number of neighbours) are more likely to be selected.

As we will show, the introduction of the parameter α yields a rich set of such networks, with an exponent β varying with α as $\beta = (3 - \alpha)/(1 - \alpha)$. In particular, if $\alpha = 0$ we obtain power-law graphs with exponent $\beta = 3$.

A descriptor of the graph $G(t)$ suitable for the identification of power laws is the following. Denote by $X_i(t)$ the number of nodes with degree i in $G(t)$. Denote by $\mathcal{F}_t$ the sigma-field containing all the information about the graphs $G(0), \ldots, G(t)$ (i.e. the node labels and the edges between them). The preferential attachment rule described above implies the following properties for the vector $X(t) = \{X_i(t)\}_{i \geq 1}$:

$$
\begin{aligned}
\mathbf{P}\left(X_1(t+1) = X_1(t) \mid \mathcal{F}_t\right) &= \alpha \frac{X_1(t)}{N(t)} + (1 - \alpha) \frac{X_1(t)}{2E(t)}, \\
\mathbf{P}\left(X_1(t+1) = X_1(t) + 1 \mid \mathcal{F}_t\right) &= 1 - \alpha \frac{X_1(t)}{N(t)} - (1 - \alpha) \frac{X_1(t)}{2E(t)}.
\end{aligned}
\tag{7.1}
$$

Similarly, for all $i > 1$, one has

$$
\begin{aligned}
\mathbf{P}(X_i(t+1) = X_i(t) + 1 \mid \mathcal{F}_t) &= \alpha \frac{X_{i-1}(t)}{N(t)} + (1 - \alpha) \frac{(i-1)X_{i-1}(t)}{2E(t)}, \\
\mathbf{P}(X_i(t+1) = X_i(t) - 1 \mid \mathcal{F}_t) &= \alpha \frac{X_i(t)}{N(t)} + (1 - \alpha) \frac{i X_i(t)}{2E(t)}, \\
\mathbf{P}(X_i(t+1) = X_i(t) \mid \mathcal{F}_t) &= 1 - \alpha \frac{X_i(t) + X_{i-1}(t)}{N(t)} - (1 - \alpha) \frac{i X_i(t) + (i-1)X_{i-1}(t)}{2E(t)}.
\end{aligned}
\tag{7.2}
$$

We now state the main result of this section.

Theorem 7.1 *Let*

$$
c_1 = \frac{2}{3 + \alpha}, \qquad \frac{c_i}{c_{i-1}} = \frac{\alpha + \frac{1-\alpha}{2}(i - 1)}{1 + \alpha + \frac{1-\alpha}{2}i}, \quad i > 1.
\tag{7.3}
$$

Then for all $i \geq 1$,

$$
\frac{X_i(t)}{t} \to c_i \text{ almost surely as } t \to \infty.
\tag{7.4}
$$

Theorem 7.1 provides a law of large number for the number of nodes with i neighbours. A consequence of the theorem is that the graph G_t is approximately a power-law random graph. Indeed, for large $i > 1$, one has

$$
\frac{c_i}{c_{i-1}} = 1 - \frac{3 - \alpha}{2 + 2\alpha + (1 - \alpha)i} = 1 - \frac{1}{i}\frac{3 - \alpha}{1 - \alpha} + O(i^{-2}).
$$

Consequently,

$$c_i = c_1 \prod_{j=2}^{i} \left(1 - \frac{1}{i}\frac{3-\alpha}{1-\alpha} + O(i^{-2}) \right) \sim A i^{-(3-\alpha)/(1-\alpha)} \text{ as } i \to \infty,$$

for some constant $A > 0$.

The proof proceeds by first controlling the average number of degree i nodes $\bar{X}_i(t) := \mathbf{E}(X_i(t))$, which is done in the next theorem.

Theorem 7.2   *For all $\epsilon > 0$, and all $i \geq 1$,*

$$\bar{X}_i(t) = c_i t + o(t^\epsilon). \tag{7.5}$$

Proof   Let $\epsilon > 0$ be fixed. Introduce the notation

$$\Delta_i(t) = \bar{X}_i(t) - c_i t, \quad i \geq 1, \, t \geq 1.$$

By equation (7.1),

$$
\begin{aligned}
\Delta_1(t+1) &= \Delta_1(t) - c_1 + 1 - \alpha \frac{\bar{X}_1}{N(t)} - (1-\alpha)\frac{\bar{X}_1(t)}{2E(t)} \\
&= \Delta_1(t)\left[1 - \frac{\alpha}{N(t)} - \frac{1-\alpha}{2E(t)} \right] - c_1 + 1 - c_1 t \left(\frac{\alpha}{N(t)} + \frac{1-\alpha}{2E(t)} \right).
\end{aligned}
$$

Note that the term $[\alpha/N(t) + (1-\alpha)/2E(t)]$ is in the interval $[0, 1]$, and furthermore it equals $t^{-1}[\alpha + (1-\alpha)/2] + O(t^{-2})$. This yields

$$
\begin{aligned}
\Delta_1(t+1) &= \Delta_1(t)\left[1 - \frac{\alpha}{N(t)} - \frac{1-\alpha}{2E(t)} \right] - c_1 + 1 - c_1(\alpha + (1-\alpha)/2) + O(t^{-1}) \\
&= \Delta_1(t)\left[1 - \frac{\alpha}{N(t)} - \frac{1-\alpha}{2E(t)} \right] + O(t^{-1}),
\end{aligned}
$$

by our choice of c_1. It thus follows that

$$|\Delta_1(t+1))| \leq |\Delta_1(t)| + O(t^{-1}) \leq O(\log(t)),$$

the latter evaluation being obtained by induction on t. Thus certainly, $\Delta_1(t) = \bar{X}_1(t) - c_1 t = o(t^\epsilon)$.

Let us now consider $i > 1$, and assume that a similar condition (7.5) holds for all $j < i$. Using (7.2), write

$$
\begin{aligned}
\Delta_i(t+1) &= \Delta_i(t) - c_i + \bar{X}_{i-1}(t)\left[\frac{\alpha}{N(t)} + \frac{(1-\alpha)(i-1)}{2E(t)} \right] - \bar{X}_i(t)\left[\frac{\alpha}{N(t)} + \frac{(1-\alpha)i}{2E(t)} \right] \\
&= -c_i + \Delta_i(t)\left[1 - \frac{\alpha}{N(t)} + \frac{(1-\alpha)i}{2E(t)} \right] + \Delta_{i-1}(t)\left[\frac{\alpha}{N(t)} + \frac{(1-\alpha)(i-1)}{2E(t)} \right] \\
&\quad + c_{i-1}t\left[1 - \frac{\alpha}{N(t)} + \frac{(1-\alpha)i}{2E(t)} \right] - c_i t \left[\frac{\alpha}{N(t)} + \frac{(1-\alpha)i}{2E(t)} \right] \\
&= \Delta_i(t)\left[1 - \frac{\alpha}{N(t)} + \frac{(1-\alpha)i}{2E(t)} \right] + O(\Delta_{i-1}(t)/t) + O(t^{-1}).
\end{aligned}
$$

By the induction hypothesis, $\Delta_{i-1}(t)/t = o(t^{\epsilon-1})$. We thus arrive at

$$|\Delta_i(t)| = o\left(\sum_{s=1}^{t} s^{\epsilon-1} \right) = o(t^\epsilon),$$

which is the claimed property. $\square$

We next need the following lemma.

Lemma 7.3 *For all $i, t \geq 1$, and all $M > 0$,*

$$\mathbf{P}\left(|X_i(t) - \bar{X}_i(t)| \geq M\right) \leq 2\exp\left(-\frac{M^2}{8t}\right). \tag{7.6}$$

Before giving the proof of this lemma, we show how, together with Theorem 7.2, it implies the result of Theorem 7.1. Take $M = 4\sqrt{t \log(t)}$ in (7.6). This yields

$$\mathbf{P}\left(|X_i(t) - \bar{X}_i(t)| \geq 4\sqrt{t \log(t)}\right) \leq 2t^{-2}.$$

The sum over $t \geq 0$ of the right-hand side $2t^{-2}$ is finite. Thus, by the Borel–Cantelli lemma, the event

$$|X_i(t) - \bar{X}_i(t)| \geq 4\sqrt{t \log(t)}$$

occurs for only finitely many t. Thus combined with Theorem 7.2, this implies that for all $\epsilon > 0$, and all large enough t,

$$|X_i(t) - c_i t| \leq t^\epsilon + 4\sqrt{t \log(t)},$$

and the result of Theorem 7.1 follows. Let us now give the proof of Lemma 7.3.

Proof Let $t, i \geq 1$ be fixed. Denote by $v(s)$ the node in $G(s-1)$ to which the node $u(s)$ attaches. We make the dependency of $X_i(t)$ on the consecutive choices $v(1), \ldots, v(t)$ explicit by writing

$$X_i(t) = f(v(1), \ldots, v(t)).$$

We further define the martingale $\{M(s)\}_{0 \leq s \leq t}$ by letting

$$M(s) = \mathbf{E}[X_i(t)|v(1), \ldots, v(s)], \quad s = 0, \ldots, t.$$

(By an elementary application of conditional probability, such processes are easily proved to be martingales.) Let us show that this martingale satisfies the following property:

$$|M(s) - M(s-1)| \leq 2 \text{ almost surely}, \quad s = 1, \ldots, t. \tag{7.7}$$

To this end, let $s \in \{1, \ldots, t\}$ be fixed. Let the sequence $v(1), \ldots, v(s)$ be given, and let another random node $V'(s)$ of $G(s-1)$ be given, which is distributed as the anchor node in $G(s)$, given that the previous anchor nodes are $v(1), \ldots, v(s-1)$. We now construct jointly random node sequences $V(s+1), \ldots, V(t)$, and $V'(s+1), \ldots, V'(t)$ with the following two properties:

- The distribution of $V(s+1), \ldots, V(t)$ (resp. $V'(s+1), \ldots, V'(t)$) is that of the $(s+1)$th to tth anchor nodes in the graph growth model under consideration, conditional on the first s anchor nodes being $v(1), \ldots, v(s)$ (resp. $v(1), \ldots, v(s-1), V'(s)$).
- Denote by $G(s), \ldots G(t)$ (resp. $G'(s), \ldots, G'(t)$) the corresponding sequence of growing graphs. For all $\ell = s, \ldots, t$, and any node u in the node set of $G(\ell)$ and $G'(\ell)$, the degree $d_\ell(u)$ of u within the graph $G(\ell)$ coincides with the degree $d'_\ell(u)$ within the graph $G'(\ell)$, unless u equals either $v(s)$ or $V'(s)$. Note that, by construction,

$$d_\ell(v(s)) + d_\ell(V'(s)) = d'_\ell(v(s)) + d'_\ell(V'(s)). \tag{7.8}$$

To perform the joint construction of the two sequences of graphs $G(s), \ldots, G(t), G'(s), \ldots, G'(t)$, we introduce a sequence of random variables $Y_{s+1}, \ldots, Y_t$ assumed i.i.d., independent of $v(1), \ldots, v(s-1), V'(s)$, taking their values in $\{0, 1\}$ and such that $\mathbf{P}(Y_\ell = 0) = \alpha$, $\ell = s+1, \ldots, t$. The random variables $Y_{s+1}, \ldots, Y_t$ correspond to indicators of whether the sampling for the anchor nodes is done uniformly or according to the preferential attachment mechanism.

The construction is then done by induction on $\ell = s+1, \ldots, t$. For any given $\ell = s+1, \ldots, t$, select the anchor nodes $V(\ell)$ and $V'(\ell)$ in $G(\ell)$ and $G'(\ell)$ respectively according to the following distribution.

- If $Y_\ell = 0$, let $V(\ell) = V'(\ell)$. This anchor node, identical for the two sequences, is selected uniformly at random from the node set of $G(\ell - 1)$, and independently of the previous random choices $V_{s+1}^{\ell-1} = (V(s+1), \ldots, V(l-1))$, $V'^{\ell-1}_s = (V'(s), \ldots, V'(\ell - 1))$ used in the joint construction so far.
- If $Y_\ell = 1$, conditional on the previous random choices, the distribution of $V(\ell), V'(\ell)$ is given by
  * if $u \notin \{v(s), V'(s)\}$,

  $$\mathbf{P}\left(V(\ell) = V'(\ell) = u \mid Y_\ell = 1, V_{s+1}^{\ell-1}, V'^{\ell-1}_s\right) = \frac{d_{\ell-1}(u)}{2E(\ell - 1)}, \tag{7.9}$$

  * if $(u, v) \in \{v(s), V'(s)\}$,

  $$\mathbf{P}\left(V(\ell) = u, V'(\ell) = v \mid Y_\ell = 1, V_{s+1}^{\ell-1}, V'^{\ell-1}_s\right)$$
  $$= \frac{d_{\ell-1}(u)d'_{\ell-1}(v)}{2E(\ell - 1)\left[d_{\ell-1}(v(s)) + d_{\ell-1}(V'(s))\right]}. \tag{7.10}$$

It is readily seen that at each step ℓ of this construction, and for each node $u \notin \{v(s), V'(s)\}$, the degrees $d_\ell(u)$ and $d'_\ell(u)$ coincide. In addition, the sequences of anchor nodes thus constructed have the desired distributions. Indeed, Formulas

(7.8)–(7.10) can be used to establish for all candidate anchor nodes u in $G(\ell-1)$ the identities

$$\mathbf{P}\left(V(\ell) = u \mid V_{s+1}^{\ell-1}, V_s'^{\ell-1}\right) = \alpha\frac{1}{N(\ell-1)} + (1-\alpha)\frac{d_{\ell-1}(u)}{2E(\ell-1)}.$$

Since the right-hand side does not depend on the conditioning sequence $V_s'^{\ell-1}$, this conditioning can be removed in this expression, which thus establishes that the anchor node $V(\ell)$ is sampled according to the desired distribution. A similar argument applies for $V'(\ell)$.

Now, Equation (7.7) follows by writing

$$|M(s) - M(s-1)| \le \left|\sum_{v_{s+1}^t, v_s'^t} \mathbf{P}(V_{s+1}^t = v_{s+1}^t, V_s'^t = v_s'^t)\left[f(v_1^t) - f(v_1^{s-1}v_s'^t)\right]\right|$$
$$\le \sum_{v_{s+1}^t, v_s'^t} \mathbf{P}(V_{s+1}^t = v_{s+1}^t, V_s'^t = v_s'^t)\left|f(v_1^t) - f(v_1^{s-1}v_s'^t)\right|.$$

However, the coupling construction ensures that in the graphs $G(t)$ and $G'(t)$, the degrees of all but at most two nodes disagree. Recall that f counts the number of degree i nodes. Then, clearly, the absolute value in the right-hand side of the equation above does not exceed 2. Since the sum of probabilities equals 1, Equation (7.7) follows. $\square$

7.3 Yule process

A precursor of the previous model is the so-called Yule process, introduced by Yule in 1925 [86] as a plausible model for the evolution of the number of species within *genera* of plants, i.e. groups of species thought to be related in some distinctive way. Yule's work provides a mathematical framework for the derivation of the distribution of such species, which had been shown empirically by Willis to satisfy a power law.

In the model, species are organised in genera. Each species gives birth, at some fixed rate, to a new species, thanks to mutations. Species do not go extinct in the basic version of the model. The new species is, with probability α, so different from any other species that it creates a new genus of its own. With the complementary probability $1 - \alpha$, it is a member of the same genus as the species from which it originates.

Denote by $X_i(t)$ the number of genera comprising exactly i species after the tth new species has appeared. The initial condition is specified by the vector $\{X_i(0)\}_{i\ge 1}$. Denoting by $\mathcal{F}_t$ the sigma-field $\sigma(X(0), \ldots, X(t))$, the dynamics is then given by

$$
\begin{aligned}
\mathbf{P}(X_1(t+1) = X_1(t) + 1 \mid \mathcal{F}_t) &= \alpha, \\
\mathbf{P}(X_1(t+1) = X_1(t) - 1 \mid \mathcal{F}_t) &= (1-\alpha)\frac{X_1(t)}{N(t)}, \\
\mathbf{P}(X_1(t+1) = X_1(t) \mid \mathcal{F}_t) &= 1 - \alpha - (1-\alpha)\frac{X_1(t)}{N(t)},
\end{aligned} \tag{7.11}
$$

where $N(t)$ denotes the total number of species. Note that

$$
N(t) = N(0) + t.
$$

Similarly, we have for all $i > 1$ and $t \geq 0$

$$
\begin{aligned}
\mathbf{P}(X_i(t+1) = X_i(t) + 1 \mid \mathcal{F}_t) &= (1-\alpha)\frac{(i-1)X_{i-1}(t)}{N(t)}, \\
\mathbf{P}(X_i(t+1) = X_i(t) - 1 \mid \mathcal{F}_t) &= (1-\alpha)\frac{iX_i(t)}{N(t)}, \\
\mathbf{P}(X_i(t+1) = X_i(t) \mid \mathcal{F}_t) &= \alpha + (1-\alpha)\left[1 - \frac{iX_i(t)+(i-1)X_{i-1}(t)}{N(t)}\right].
\end{aligned} \tag{7.12}
$$

We now establish the following result about the number of genera of different sizes that we expect to see in the long run.

Theorem 7.4 *Let*

$$
c_1 = \frac{\alpha}{2-\alpha}, \quad \frac{c_i}{c_{i-1}} = 1 - \frac{2-\alpha}{1+i(1-\alpha)}, \; i > 1. \tag{7.13}
$$

Then for all $i \geq 1$,

$$
\frac{X_i(t)}{t} \to c_i \text{ almost surely as } t \to \infty. \tag{7.14}
$$

The proof proceeds along the same lines as that of Theorem 7.1. We first analyse the asymptotic behaviour of the expected values $\bar{X}_i(t) := \mathbf{E}(X_i(t))$.

Theorem 7.5 *For all $\epsilon > 0$, and all $i \geq 1$,*

$$
\bar{X}_i(t) = c_i t + o(t^\epsilon). \tag{7.15}
$$

Proof Define as before $\Delta_i(t) = \bar{X}_i(t) - c_i t$, for all $i, t \geq 1$. For $i = 1$, we have

$$
\begin{aligned}
\Delta_1(t+1) &= \Delta_1(t) - c_1 + \alpha - (1-\alpha)\frac{\bar{X}_1(t)}{N(t)} \\
&= \Delta_1(t)\left(1 - \frac{1-\alpha}{N(t)}\right) - c_1 + \alpha - (1-\alpha)\frac{c_1 t}{N(t)} \\
&= \Delta_1(t)\left(1 - \frac{1-\alpha}{N(t)}\right) + O(t^{-1}),
\end{aligned}
$$

which again ensures that $\Delta_1(t) = O(\log(t))$.

Let us assume that for all $j < i$ and all $\epsilon > 0$, $\Delta_j(t) = o(t^\epsilon)$. Then write

$$
\begin{aligned}
\Delta_i(t+1) &= \Delta_i(t) - c_i + \frac{1-\alpha}{N(t)}\left[(i-1)\bar{X}_{i-1}(t) - i\bar{X}_i(t)\right] \\
&= \Delta_i(t)\left[1 - \frac{(1-\alpha)i}{N(t)}\right] + \frac{(1-\alpha)(i-1)}{N(t)}\Delta_{i-1}(t) \\
&\quad - c_i\left(1 + \frac{(1-\alpha)it}{N(t)}\right) + c_{i-1}\frac{(1-\alpha)(i-1)t}{N(t)} \\
&= \Delta_i(t)\left[1 - \frac{(1-\alpha)i}{N(t)}\right] + O(t^{\epsilon-1}),
\end{aligned}
$$

where we have used the induction assumption $\Delta_{i-1}(t) = o(t^\epsilon)$, and cancellation of terms based on the expression for c_i/c_{i-1} in (7.13). The result (7.15) easily follows. □

In order to conclude the proof of Theorem 7.4, let us establish that the statement of Lemma 7.3 is true with the state variables $X_i(t)$ for the Yule process rather than for the preferential attachment graph. Let i, t be fixed. Denote by $v(s)$ the label of the species that gave birth to a new species at the sth such birth, and let $\xi_s \in \{0, 1\}$ equal 1 if this new species starts a new genus, and 0 otherwise. Denote by $x(s)$ the pair $(v(s), \xi_s)$. Note that the variables $\{x(s)\}_{s=1,\ldots,t}$ are independent, $v(s)$ being uniform on the label set of species at time $s - 1$ (for definiteness, take the label set to be $\{1, \ldots, N(s - 1)\}$) and independent of ξ_s, which is a Bernoulli random variable equal to 1 with probability α. Writing

$$X_i(t) = f(x(1), \ldots, x(t))$$

we now show that we can use the second form of the Azuma–Hoeffding inequality, Corollary 6.4, to control the deviations of this random variable from its mean. Indeed, consider a sequence $x_1^t = (x_1, \ldots, x_t)$, and another sequence $x_1^{s-1} y_s x_{s+1}^t$ differing from the first only in its sth coordinate. Look at a graphical representation in which a new species is identified with a graph node and is connected to its generating species by an edge if it belongs to the same genus, and to no other genus otherwise (see Figure 7.1). By changing the coordinate x_s to y_s in the sequence x_1^t we are simply modifying the endpoint of the edge connecting the sth node to the older part of the graph: we may either remove this edge, or create it if it was absent. The number of genera consisting of i species is exactly the number of connected components with i nodes in the graphical representation.

Removing one edge of a graph may split a connected component into two. This removes at most one connected component of size i and creates at most two connected components of size i. Thus addition/removal of one edge modifies the number of size i components by at most 2.

Similarly, changing the endpoint of one edge removes at most two size i components. By symmetry, it adds at most two such components. This shows that, for the function f that counts the number of size i genera,

$$\left| f(x_1^t) - f(x_1^{s-1} y_s x_{s+1}^t) \right| \le 2 \,,$$

for all possible choices of x_1^t, $s = 1, \ldots, t$, and y_s. Thus Corollary 6.4 applies, and the proof of Theorem 7.4 then parallels that of Theorem 7.1.

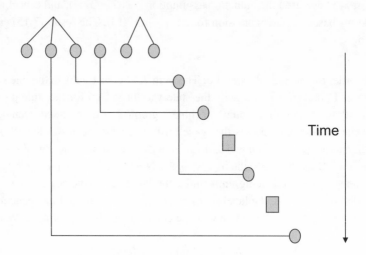

Time

Figure 7.1 Graphical representation of the Yule process. A square is a species
starting a new genus; a circle is a species connected to its originating species,
hence part of the same genus.

7.4 Notes

Both power-law graphs and the Yule process describe models of networks
where the degree distribution exhibits heterogeneous statistics in contrast with
network models such as E-R random graphs, de Bruijn graphs and small-world
graphs. They represent a benchmark for such heterogeneous statistics. In the
next chapter we will analyse the outcome of an epidemic on homogeneous
networks such as the E-R graph and heterogeneous networks exemplified by
power-law networks and pinpoint the impact of the statistics of the degree distribution on the spread of an epidemic.

For further reading: Mitzenmacher [66] discusses other models for generating power laws, as well as log-normal distributions. He also reviews a jus-
tification completely different from the preferential attachment model, due to
Mandelbrot [62], for the fact that the distribution of word occurences in a text
follows a power law. According to Mandelbrot, such power laws yield the maximal information rate per length of text, counted in letters rather than words.

A richer model than that of Barabási-Albert, featuring multiple edge addi-
tions per node arrival and oriented edges, is presented in Bollobás *et al.* [14],
together with an analysis of the resulting power laws for both in-degrees and
out-degrees.

8

Epidemics on general graphs

8.1 Introduction

In this chapter we investigate the behaviour of two classical epidemic models on general graphs. We consider a closed population of n individuals, connected by a neighbourhood structure that is represented by an undirected, labelled graph $G = (V, E)$ with node set $V = \{1, \ldots, n\}$ and edge set E. Each node can be in one of three possible states: susceptible (S), infective (I) or removed (R). The initial set of infectives at time 0 is assumed to be non empty, and all other nodes are assumed to be susceptible at time 0. We will focus on two classical epidemic models: the susceptible-infected-removed (SIR) and susceptible-infected-susceptible (SIS) epidemic processes.

In what follows we represent the graph by means of its adjacency matrix A, i.e. $a_{ij} = 1$ if $(i, j) \in E$ and $a_{ij} = 0$ otherwise. Since the graph G is undirected, A is a symmetric, non-negative matrix, all its eigenvalues are real, the eigenvalue with the largest absolute value ρ is positive and its associated eigenvector has non-negative entries (by the Perron–Frobenius theorem). The value ρ is called the *spectral radius*. If the graph is connected, as we shall assume, then this eigenvalue has multiplicity one, the corresponding eigenvector is strictly positive and is the only one with all elements non-negative. For the two models of interest we will answer the following questions: What impact does the topology have on the speed of spread of the epidemic, and moreover what are the key features of the topology that determine how virulent the epidemic is? In particular we will show the existence of epidemic thresholds that are related to the spectrum of the graph's adjacency matrix.

8.2 Reed–Frost model

The first model is the Reed-Frost model, a particular example of an SIR epidemic process, introduced in Chapter 2. The evolution of the epidemic is described by the following discrete-time model. Let $X_v(t)$ denote the indicator that node v is infected at the beginning of time slot t and $Y_v(t)$ the indicator that it has been removed. Each node that is infected at the beginning of a time slot attempts to infect each of its neighbours; each infection attempt is successful with probability β independent of other infection attempts. Each infected node is removed at the end of the time slot. Thus, the probability that a susceptible node u becomes infected at the end of time slot t is given by $1 - \prod_{v \sim u}(1 - \beta X_v(t))$, where we write $v \sim u$ to mean that $(u, v) \in E$. Note that the evolution stops when there are no more infectives in the population.

The object of interest is the number of nodes that eventually become infected (and removed) compared to the number initially infected. As established in Chapter 2, Theorem 2.1, the number of nodes infected in the Reed–Frost model on the complete graph exhibits a sharp threshold as the infection probability is increased; it jumps suddenly from a negligible to a non-zero fraction of n, the number of nodes in the system. We wish to ask if a similar threshold phenomenon occurs on general graphs and, if so, how the critical value of β is related to properties of the graph.

We will denote by $|X(t)| = \sum_{i=1}^{n} X_i(t)$ and $|Y(t)| = \sum_{i=1}^{n} Y_i(t)$ the number of infected and removed individuals at time t, respectively. Similarly we define $|Y(\infty)|$ as the number of nodes that are eventually removed.

Theorem 8.1 *Suppose $\beta\rho < 1$, where ρ is the spectral radius of the adjacency matrix A. Then the total number $|Y(\infty)|$ of nodes removed satisfies*

$$\mathbf{E}\left[|Y(\infty)|\right] \le \frac{1}{1 - \beta\rho} \sqrt{n|X(0)|},$$

where $|X(0)|$ is the number of initial infectives.

If the graph G is regular (i.e. each node has the same number of neighbours) with node degree d, then

$$\mathbf{E}\left[|Y(\infty)|\right] \le \frac{1}{1 - \beta\rho}|X(0)| = \frac{1}{1 - \beta d}|X(0)|.$$

Proof In order for an arbitrary node v to be infected at the start of time slot t, there must be a chain of distinct nodes $u_0, u_1, \ldots, u_t = v$ along which the infection passes from some initial infective u_0 to v. Thus, by the union bound,

$$\mathbf{P}(X_v(t) = 1) \le \sum_{u_0, \ldots, u_{t-1}} \beta^t X_{u_0}(0),$$

where the sum is taken over nodes $u_0, \ldots, u_{t-1}$ such that $(u_{i-1}, u_i) \in E$ for all $i = 1, \ldots, t$, where we take $u_t = v$. Note that we have not imposed the requirement that the u_i be distinct as we are only seeking an upper bound. Consequently, the probability that node v ever gets infected (and hence that $Y_v(\infty) = 1$) is bounded above by

$$\mathbf{P}(Y_v(\infty) = 1) \le \sum_{t=0}^{\infty} \sum_{u \in V} (\beta A)_{uv}^t X_u(0),$$

since the uvth entry of the matrix A^t is simply the number of paths of length t between nodes u and v. It is immediate from the above that

$$\mathbf{E}[|Y(\infty)|] = \sum_{v \in V} \mathbf{P}(Y_v(\infty) = 1) \le \sum_{t=0}^{\infty} e^T (\beta A)^t X(0),$$

where e denotes the vector of ones. If $\beta \rho < 1$, then we can rewrite the above as

$$\mathbf{E}[|Y(\infty)|] \le e^T (I - \beta A)^{-1} X(0)$$
$$\le \|e\| \left\| (I - \beta A)^{-1} \right\| \|X(0)\|, \tag{8.1}$$

where $\|\cdot\|$ denotes the Euclidean norm in the case of a vector, and the matrix or operator norm in the case of a matrix. Now the operator norm of a symmetric matrix is its spectral radius, the largest of its eigenvalues in absolute value. Hence $\left\| (I - \beta A)^{-1} \right\| = (1 - \beta \rho)^{-1}$. Moreover, $\|X(0)\| = \sqrt{\sum_{v \in V} X_v^2(0)} = \sqrt{|X(0)|}$. Likewise, $\|\mathbf{1}\| = \sqrt{n}$. Substituting these in (8.1) yields

$$\mathbf{E}[|Y(\infty)|] \le \frac{1}{1 - \beta \rho} \sqrt{n|X(0)|},$$

which is the first claim of the theorem.

Next, note that by using the spectral decomposition

$$(I - \beta A)^{-1} = \sum_{i=1}^{n} \frac{1}{1 - \beta \lambda_i} x_i x_i^T,$$

where x_i denotes the eigenvector corresponding to the eigenvalue λ_i of A, and x_i^T its transpose, we can rewrite (8.1) as

$$\mathbf{E}[|Y(\infty)|] \le \sum_{i=1}^{n} \frac{1}{1 - \beta \lambda_i} e^T x_i x_i^T X(0). \tag{8.2}$$

If G is a regular graph and each node has degree d (i.e. has exactly d neighbours), then each row sum of its adjacency matrix A is equal to d. Hence, it is clear that the positive vector $\frac{1}{\sqrt{n}} e$ is an eigenvector of A corresponding to the eigenvalue d. By the Perron–Frobenius theorem, this is therefore the largest eigenvalue. Hence, $\lambda_1 = \rho = d$, $x_1 = \frac{1}{\sqrt{n}}e$, and all other eigenvectors $x_2, \ldots, x_n$ are orthogonal to e. Hence, by (8.2),

$$\mathbf{E}\left[|Y(\infty)|\right] \le \frac{1}{1 - \beta\rho} e^T x_1 x_1^T X(0)$$

$$= \frac{1}{n(1 - \beta d)} e^T e e^T X(0) = \frac{1}{1 - \beta d} |X(0)|.$$

This is the second claim of the theorem. □

The theorem says that, if $\beta\rho < 1$, then starting from a "small" population of initial infectives, the final size of the epidemic is small. For example, if $|X(0)| = 1$, then the final size of the epidemic is bounded by a constant in the case of regular graphs, and by a multiple of $\sqrt{n}$ in general. Thus, the fraction of nodes infected goes to zero as n tends to infinity. The upper bounds in the theorem are close to the best possible in general, as we will see later when we consider the star-shaped network.

8.3 SIS model

We now consider the susceptible-infected-susceptible (SIS) model, also known as the contact process. It is described as follows. A graph G is given, with a finite node set $\{1, \ldots, n\}$. The variable $X_i(t)$ tracks the health status of node i: it is infected if $X_i(t) = 1$, and healthy if $X_i(t) = 0$. Infected nodes return to the susceptible state at unit rate, while susceptible nodes become infected at a rate that is the product of the base infection rate, $\beta > 0$, and the number of graph neighbours that are infected.

Such dynamics could be plausible models of the following situations:

- epidemics of mutating viruses, where a new mutant can re-infect an individual previously infected by another version of the virus (think of influenza);
- a crude information storage system. Here, nodes correspond to storage locations; they remove stored information at unit rate, while nodes holding some information replicate it at neighbour nodes at some rate β.

In these two scenarios, a quantity of interest is the time to recovery from the epidemic (in the second situation, this would correspond to information loss by the system). Note that, when the graph is finite, extinction of the epidemic is inevitable. This is in contrast with the case of infinite graphs, where infection can survive forever. For a survey of results for the contact process on infinite graphs, such as regular grids and trees, see [57].

A more formal description of the contact process is as follows. It is a Markov jump process on $\{0, 1\}^n$, with non-zero transition rates $q(x, y)$ between states $x, y \in \{0, 1\}^n$ given by

$$
\begin{aligned}
q(x, x + e_i) &= \beta(1 - x_i) \sum_{j \sim i} x_j, \quad x \in \{0, 1\}^n, \ i \in \{1, \ldots, n\}, \\
q(x, x - e_i) &= x_i, \quad x \in \{0, 1\}^n, \ i \in \{1, \ldots, n\}.
\end{aligned}
\tag{8.3}
$$

In (8.3), $i \sim j$ means that i and j are graph neighbours, and e_i denotes the vector with its ith coordinate equal to 1, and all other coordinates equal to 0.

We first give a sufficient condition for fast extinction (absorption at 0) of the process. We then give a sufficient condition for long survival of the process.

8.3.1 Fast extinction and spectral radius for the SIS epidemics

Recall that the adjacency matrix A of a graph G is determined by $A_{ij} = 1$ if $i \sim j$, and 0 otherwise. Also recall that the spectral radius of a matrix is the maximum of the absolute value of its eigenvalues. We shall establish the following.

Theorem 8.2 *Let A denote the adjacency matrix of graph G, and ρ denote the spectral radius of this matrix. Then for any initial condition $X(0) = \{X_i(0)\}_{i=1,\ldots,n}$, and all $t \geq 0$, one has the following:*

$$
\mathbf{P}(X(t) \neq 0) \leq \sqrt{n \sum_{i=1}^{n} X_i(0)} \exp((\beta \rho - 1)t) ,
\tag{8.4}
$$

where $X(t) := \{X_i(t)\}_{i=1,\ldots,n}$ denotes the state of the contact process with parameter β, on graph G, at time t.

In order to establish this result, we shall rely on a general coupling technique, which allows us to relate the trajectories of different Markov processes. This will be phrased in the context of skip-free Markov jump processes, which we now define.

Definition 8.3 (Skip-free Markov jump process)   Let $K > 0$ be some fixed integer. A *skip-free Markov jump process* on the state $\mathbb{N}^K$ is by definition a Markov jump process on this state space, whose transition rates $q(x, y)$, for $x \neq y \in \mathbb{N}^K$, are all zero except when $y = x + e_i$ or $y = x - e_i$ for some $i \in \{1, \ldots, K\}$. The transition rate $q(x, x + e_i)$ is also referred to as the birth rate at site i when in state x. Similarly, the transition rate $q(x, x - e_i)$ is the death rate at site i when in state x.

The basic coupling result we shall use is the following.

Theorem 8.4   *Consider two skip-free Markov jump processes X, X′ defined on the state space $\mathbb{N}^K$, with respective birth rates $\beta_i(x)$, $\beta_i'(x)$ and death rates $\delta_i(x)$, $\delta_i'(x)$, for $x \in \mathbb{N}^K$ and $i \in \{1, \ldots, K\}$.*

Assume that for all $x, y \in \mathbb{N}^K$ such that $x \leq y$ (i.e. $x_i \leq y_i$ for all $i = \{1, \ldots, K\}$), the following holds:

$$x_i = y_i \Rightarrow \beta_i(x) \leq \beta_i'(y) \text{ and } \delta_i(x) \geq \delta_i'(y). \tag{8.5}$$

Then, for initial conditions $X(0)$ and $X'(0)$ satisfying $X(0) \leq X'(0)$, one can construct the two processes X, X′ jointly so that for all $t \geq 0$, the ordering is preserved, that is $X(t) \leq X'(t)$.

Proof   Consider the Markov process on the state space $\{(x, x') \in \mathbb{N}^K \times \mathbb{N}^K : x \leq x'\}$, with only non-zero transition rates given as follows. For any state (x, x') and $i \in \{1, \ldots, K\}$, if $x_i < x_i'$ the non-zero transition rates are

$$\begin{aligned}
q((x, x'), (x + e_i, x')) &= \beta_i(x)\,, \\
q((x, x'), (x, x' + e_i)) &= \beta_i'(x')\,, \\
q((x, x'), (x - e_i, x')) &= \delta_i(x)\,, \\
q((x, x'), (x, x' - e_i)) &= \delta_i'(x')\,.
\end{aligned} \tag{8.6}$$

When $x_i = x_i'$, the non-zero transition rates are given by

$$\begin{aligned}
q((x, x'), (x + e_i, x' + e_i)) &= \beta_i(x)\,, \\
q((x, x'), (x, x' + e_i)) &= \beta_i'(x') - \beta_i(x)\,, \\
q((x, x'), (x - e_i, x' - e_i)) &= \delta_i'(x')\,, \\
q((x, x'), (x - e_i, x')) &= \delta_i(x) - \delta_i'(x')\,.
\end{aligned} \tag{8.7}$$

Note that these terms are non-negative when condition (8.5) holds. The proof of Theorem 8.4 will be concluded by establishing that the Markov process $(X(t), X'(t))_{t>0}$ started from initial condition $(X(0), X'(0))$ and whose dynamics are specified by these transition rates is such that the component processes $(X(t))_{t>0}$ and $(X'(t))_{t>0}$ are skip-free Markov jump processes with the desired birth and death rates given by the functions (β, δ) and (β', δ') respectively. Since by construction, $X(t) \leq X'(t)$ for all $t > 0$, the result will follow.

To establish that the component processes indeed have the desired dynamics, we use the following result.

Lemma 8.5   *Let a Markov jump process $\{Y(t)\}_{t \geq 0}$ on a countable state space E, with transition rates $q(x, y)$, $x, y \in E$, and let a function $f : E \to F$ be given, where F is another countable state space. Assume that there exists a function $\tilde{q}(u, v)$ defined on $F \times F$ such that, for all $i \in E$ and all $v \in F$, one has*

$$\sum_{j : f(j) = v} q(i, j) = \tilde{q}(f(i), v). \tag{8.8}$$

Then the image process $Z(t) := f(Y(t))$ is a Markov jump process on F, with transition rates $\tilde{q}(u, v)$.

Proof We first prove the analogous result for discrete-time Markov chains. Let $(X_k)_{k \in \mathbb{N}}$ be a Markov chain with transition matrix $P = (p(x, y))_{x,y \in \mathbb{N}}$ and $Y_k = f(X_k)$, where the function f is such that there exists a transition matrix $\tilde{P}$ satisfying

$$\sum_{y: f(y) = v} p(x, y) = \tilde{p}(f(x), v) . \tag{8.9}$$

To prove the lemma in this discrete-time setup, write

$$\mathbf{P}(Y_1 = y_1, \ldots, Y_k = y_k \mid Y_0 = y_0) = \frac{\displaystyle\sum_{x_i, f(x_i) = y_i, \, i=0,\ldots,k} \mathbf{P}(X_0 = x_0, \ldots, X_k = x_k)}{\displaystyle\sum_{x_0, f(x_0) = y_0} \mathbf{P}(X_0 = x_0)}$$

$$= \frac{\displaystyle\sum_{x_i, f(x_i) = y_i \, i=0,\ldots,k} \mathbf{P}(X_0 = x_0) \prod_{i=0}^{k-1} p(x_i, x_{i+1})}{\displaystyle\sum_{x_0, f(x_0) = y_0} \mathbf{P}(X_0 = x_0)} .$$

Note that, in view of assumption (8.9), $\sum_{x_k, f(x_k) = y_k} p(x_{k-1}, x_k) = \tilde{p}(y_{k-1}, y_k)$. It easily follows by induction that

$$\mathbf{P}(Y_1 = y_1, \cdots, Y_k = y_k \mid Y_0 = y_0) = \prod_{i=0}^{k-1} \tilde{p}(y_i, y_{i+1}) .$$

Thus, the image process $\{Y_k\}_{k \geq 0}$ is a Markov chain with transition matrix $\tilde{P}$.

The continuous-time version is more intricate, as the image jump process $Z(t) = f(Y(t))$ may stay in the same state z whereas the process $Y(t)$ jumps between states y_i such that $f(y_i) = z$. We analyse the behaviour of the discrete-time embedded Markov chain $(Z_k)_{k \geq 0}$ keeping track of the states visited by process $\{Z(t)\}_{t \geq 0}$.

We prove the result for the first jump; the general case follows using the same ideas. Let Y_k be the discrete-time embedded Markov chain of $Y(t)$ and τ_0 the time spent by $Z(t)$ in its initial state. We are interested in evaluating

$$\mathbf{E}\left(e^{-\alpha \tau_0} \mathbf{1}_{\{Z_1 = z_1, \, Z_0 = z_0\}}\right)$$

$$= \sum_{n \geq 1} \sum_{i=0}^{n-1} \sum_{f(y_i) = z_0} \mathbf{P}(Y_0 = y_0) \sum_{f(y_n) = z_1} \prod_{i=0}^{n-1} \left(\frac{q(y_i, y_{i+1})}{q(y_i)}\right) \prod_{i=0}^{n-1} \left(\frac{q(y_i)}{q(y_i) + \alpha}\right)$$

$$\text{where } q(y_i) = \sum_{y \neq y_i} q(y_i, y).$$

Note that, for y_i such that $f(y_i) = z_0$, we have

$$
\begin{aligned}
q(y_i) = \sum_{y' \neq y_i} q(y_i, y') &= \sum_{z \in F} \sum_{y', f(y')=z} q(y_i, y') \\
&= \sum_{z \in F} \tilde{q}(z_0, z) \\
&= \tilde{q}(z_0, z_0) + \sum_{z \neq z_0} \tilde{q}(z_0, z) \\
&= \tilde{q}(z_0, z_0) + \tilde{q}(z_0) ,
\end{aligned}
$$

where $\tilde{q}(z_0) = \sum_{z \neq z_0} \tilde{q}(z_0, z)$. Dividing the sum into two parts, according to whether $n = 0$ or $n > 0$, it is not difficult to check that

$$
\mathbf{E}\left(e^{-\alpha \tau_0} \mathbf{1}_{\{Z_1 = z_1, Z_0 = z_0\}}\right) = \sum_{f(y_0)=z_0} \mathbf{P}(Y_0 = y_0) \frac{\tilde{q}(z_0, z_1)}{\tilde{q}(z_0) + \tilde{q}(z_0, z_0) + \alpha}
$$

$$
+ \mathbf{E}\left(e^{-\alpha \tau_0} \mathbf{1}_{\{Z_1 = z_1, Z_0 = z_0\}}\right) \frac{\tilde{q}(z_0, z_0)}{\tilde{q}(z_0, z_0) + \tilde{q}(z_0) + \alpha} .
$$

Thus

$$
\mathbf{E}\left(e^{-\alpha \tau_0} \mathbf{1}_{Z_1 = z_1} \mid Z_0 = z_0\right) = \frac{\tilde{q}(z_0, z_1)}{\tilde{q}(z_0) + \alpha} .
$$

The joint distribution of the next state visited after state z_0 and the sojourn time distribution in state z_0 corresponds to a Markov jump process with infinitesimal generator $\tilde{q}$.[1] Similar calculations apply to an arbitrary sequence of visited states and corresponding sojourn times. □

Let us now use this result to show that the components of the above-defined coupled process have the desired dynamics. Let $f : \mathbb{N}^K \times \mathbb{N}^K \to \mathbb{N}^K$ be defined by $f(x, x') = x$.

For any x, and any $x' \geq x$, and any $y \in \mathbb{N}^K$, we need to check the following identity:

$$
\sum_{z \in \mathbb{N}^K} q((x, x'), (y, z)) = \begin{cases} \beta_i(x) & \text{if } y = x + e_i, \\ \delta_i(x) & \text{if } y = x - e_i, \\ 0 & \text{otherwise.} \end{cases}
$$

This is easily verified from the rate specifications (8.6) and (8.7). The same needs to be done for the second component; again this is straightforward. □

We now return to the proof of Theorem 8.2. Define the so-called *branching random walk* process on $\mathbb{N}^n$ as the skip-free Markov jump process with birth

---

[1] The *sojourn time* is the time spent by the Markov chain in state z_0.

and death rates

$$\beta_i^{\mathrm{brw}}(x) = \beta \sum_{j\sim i} x_j, \quad \delta_i^{\mathrm{brw}}(x) = x_i, \ i \in \{1, \ldots, n\}.$$

Also, view the contact process as a skip-free Markov jump process on $\mathbb{N}^n$, by extending the definition of its birth and death rates $\beta^{\mathrm{c}}, \delta^{\mathrm{c}}$ to $\mathbb{N}^n$ as follows:

$$\beta_i^{\mathrm{c}}(x) = \mathbf{1}_{x_i=0}\beta \sum_{j\sim i} x_j, \quad \delta_i^{\mathrm{c}}(x) = x_i, \ i \in \{1, \ldots, n\}.$$

Next, we verify that the branching random walk and the contact process thus defined satisfy the assumptions of Theorem 8.4. To this end, let $x \leq x'$, and let i be such that $x_i = x'_i$. For all such parameter choices, we need to verify

$$\delta_i^{\mathrm{c}}(x) \geq \delta_i^{\mathrm{brw}}(x').$$

This holds trivially, as the two terms equal x_i. It only remains to check that

$$\beta_i^{\mathrm{c}}(x) \leq \beta_i^{\mathrm{brw}}(x').$$

The left-hand side is less than $\beta \sum_{j\sim i} x_j$, which is clearly less than $\beta \sum_{j\sim i} x'_j = \beta_i^{\mathrm{brw}}(x')$ when $x \leq x'$. Theorem 8.4 thus applies.

Using the coupled construction of the two processes $(X^{\mathrm{c}}(t), X^{\mathrm{brw}}(t))_{t\geq 0}$, started from the same initial condition $X(0) \in \{0, 1\}^n$, provided by this theorem, write

$$\begin{aligned} \mathbf{P}(X^{\mathrm{c}}(t) \neq 0) &\leq \mathbf{P}(X^{\mathrm{brw}}(t) \neq 0) \\ &\leq e^T \mathbf{E}(X^{\mathrm{brw}}(t)). \end{aligned}$$

The linear structure of the transition rates of the branching random walk implies that

$$\frac{d}{dt}\mathbf{E}\left(X^{\mathrm{brw}}(t)\right) = \beta A \, \mathbf{E}\left(X^{\mathrm{brw}}(t)\right) - \mathbf{E}\left(X^{\mathrm{brw}}(t)\right),$$

which solves to give

$$\mathbf{E}\left(X^{\mathrm{brw}}(t)\right) = \exp\left(t(\beta A - I)\right) X(0),$$

where I is the identity matrix, A the adjacency matrix of G and $\exp(t(\beta A - I))$ the matrix exponential of the matrix $t(\beta A - I)$. We thus have

$$\mathbf{P}(X^{\mathrm{c}}(t) \neq 0) \leq e^T \exp\left(t(\beta A - I)\right) X(0),$$

where $e = (1, \ldots, 1)^T$. By the Cauchy–Schwarz inequality, the right-hand side of the inequality above is not larger than

$$\|e\| \times \left\|\exp\left(t(\beta A - I)\right) X(0)\right\|.$$

However, since the matrix involved in the second term is symmetric, this term is not larger than $\|X(0)\|$ times the spectral radius of this matrix. The latter equals $\exp((\beta\rho - 1)t)$, which thus yields

$$\mathbf{P}(X^c(t) \neq 0) \leq \|e\| \exp((\beta\rho - 1)t)\|X(0)\|$$

$$= \sqrt{n \sum_{i=1}^{n} X_i^2(0) \exp((\beta\rho - 1)t)}$$

$$= \sqrt{n \sum_{i=1}^{n} X_i(0) \exp((\beta\rho - 1)t)} ,$$

which is the claimed result. The last equality holds because $X_i^2(0) = X_i(0)$, since $X_i(0) \in \{0, 1\}$.

The main application of Theorem 8.2 is the following corollary.

Corollary 8.6 *Consider the contact process on a finite graph G on n nodes, with base infection rate β and arbitrary initial condition $X(0) \in \{0, 1\}^n$. Let τ denote the time to absorption at 0 by the process. Then, under the condition*

$$\beta\rho < 1 , \tag{8.10}$$

where ρ is the spectral radius of the adjacency matrix of G, it holds that

$$\mathbf{E}(\tau) \leq \frac{\log n + 1}{1 - \beta\rho} . \tag{8.11}$$

Proof Write

$$\mathbf{E}(\tau) = \int_0^\infty \mathbf{P}(\tau > 0) \, dt$$

$$= \int_0^\infty \mathbf{P}(X(t) \neq 0) \, dt$$

$$\leq \int_0^\infty \min(1, n \exp(-(1 - \beta\rho)t)) \, dt$$

$$= t^* + \int_{t^*}^\infty n \exp(-(1 - \beta\rho)t) \, dt,$$

where $t^* = (\log n)/(1 - \beta\rho)$. We thus obtain

$$\mathbf{E}(\tau) \leq t^* + \frac{n}{1 - \beta\rho} \exp(-(1 - \beta\rho)t^*) = \frac{\log n + 1}{1 - \beta\rho} .$$

$\square$

8.3.2 Long survival and isoperimetric constants

We now provide a sufficient condition for long survival of the epidemics. This is phrased in terms of the isoperimetric constant of the supporting graph, which we now define.

Definition 8.7 (Isoperimetric constant)   For a graph G on the node set $\{1,\ldots,n\}$, and any integer $m < n$, the *isoperimetric constant* $\eta(m)$ of graph G is defined by

$$\eta(m) = \min_{S \subset \{1,\ldots,n\}, |S| \leq m} \frac{E(S, \bar{S})}{|S|}, \qquad (8.12)$$

where $\bar{S}$ denotes the complementary set $\{1,\ldots,n\} \setminus S$, and $E(S, T)$ denotes the number of edges with one endpoint in set S and the other in set T.

The main result of this section is the following.

Theorem 8.8   *Let a finite graph G on n nodes be given, and assume that for some $m < n$ and some $r \in (0, 1)$, it holds that*

$$\beta\eta(m) \geq \frac{1}{r}, \qquad (8.13)$$

where $\eta(m)$ denotes the isoperimetric constant of G. Then, denoting by τ the time to absorption of the contact process on G, for any initial condition $X(0) \neq 0$, it holds that:

$$\mathbf{P}\left(\tau \geq \frac{s}{2m}\right) \geq \frac{1-r}{1-r^m}\left(\frac{1-r^{m-1}}{1-r^m}\right)^s \left(1 - o(s^{-1})\right), \quad s \in \mathbb{N}, \qquad (8.14)$$

where the term $o(s^{-1})$ is independent of the model parameters.

Proof   Consider the Markov jump process $\{Z(t)\}_{t \geq 0}$ defined on the state space $\{0,\ldots,m\}$, with non-zero transition rates

$$\begin{aligned} q(z, z+1) &= r^{-1}z\mathbf{1}_{z<m}, \ z \in \{0,\ldots,m\}, \\ q(z, z-1) &= z, \ z \in \{0,\ldots,m\}. \end{aligned}$$

We now show that for any initial condition $X(0) \neq 0$, the contact process on G can be coupled with the process $\{Z(t)\}_{t \geq 0}$ with initial condition $Z(0) = 1$, in such a way that $\sum_{i=1}^{n} X_i(t) \geq Z(t)$ for all $t \geq 0$. To this end, we define the joint process (X, Z) on the state space $\{(x, z) \in \{0,1\}^n \times \{0,\ldots,m\}, z \leq \sum_{i=1}^{n} x_i\}$ as follows. For any state (x, z) and any $i \in \{1,\ldots,n\}$, if $\sum_{i=1}^{n} x_i > z$, we have the non-zero transition rates

$$\begin{aligned} q((x,z), (x+e_i, z)) &= \beta(1 - x_i)\sum_{j \sim i} x_j, \\ q((x,z), (x-e_i, z)) &= x_i, \\ q((x,z), (x, z+1)) &= r^{-1}z\mathbf{1}_{z<m}, \\ q((x,z), (x, z-1)) &= z. \end{aligned}$$

If $\sum_{i=1}^{n} x_i = z$, the non-zero transition rates are

$$q((x, z), (x + e_i, z + 1)) \quad = c_i(x),$$
$$q((x, z), (x + e_i, z)) \qquad = \beta(1 - x_i) \sum_{j \sim i} x_j - c_i(x),$$
$$q((x, z), (x - e_i, z - 1)) \quad = x_i,$$

where the rates $c_i(x)$ are chosen to satisfy the following conditions:

$$0 \le c_i(x) \le \beta(1 - x_i) \sum_{j \sim i} x_j, \ i \in \{1, \dots, n\},$$

which ensures that the transition rates are non-negative, and

$$\sum_{i=1}^{n} c_i(x) = r^{-1} z \mathbf{1}_{z<m}.$$

Let us show that such rates $c_i(x)$ exist. This will be the case if we have

$$\sum_{i=1}^{n} \beta(1 - x_i) \sum_{j \sim i} x_j \ge r^{-1} z \mathbf{1}_{z<m}.$$

Note now that the left-hand side of this equation also reads $\beta E(S, \bar{S})$, where S denotes the set of sites $j \in \{1, \dots, n\}$ such that $x_j = 1$. Note also that $|S| = \sum_j x_j = z \le m$; hence, by the definition of the isoperimetric constant $\eta(m)$, the left-hand side is greater than or equal to $\beta \eta z$. In view of condition (8.13), this is indeed larger than z/r.

One can then easily verify that the component processes have the desired dynamics by checking that Lemma 8.5 applies. This coupling implies that

$$\mathbf{P}(\tau > s) \ge \mathbf{P}(Z(s) = 0). \tag{8.15}$$

To evaluate the right-hand side of inequality (8.15), consider the discrete-time embedded Markov chain $\{Y(k)\}_{k \ge 0}$ keeping track of the states visited by process $\{Z(t)\}_{t \ge 0}$. Its non-zero transition probabilities are given by

$$\mathbf{P}(Y(k + 1) = y + 1 \mid Y(k) = y) \quad = \frac{y/r}{y/r + y} = \frac{1}{1 + r}, \ y \in \{1, \dots, m - 1\},$$
$$\mathbf{P}(Y(k + 1) = y - 1 \mid Y(k) = y) \quad = \frac{y}{y/r + y} = \frac{r}{r + 1}, \ y \in \{1, \dots, m - 1\},$$
$$\mathbf{P}(Y(k + 1) = m - 1 \mid Y(k) = m) \quad = 1,$$
$$\mathbf{P}(Y(k + 1) = 0 \mid Y(k) = 0) \qquad = 1.$$

The probability π_k that, starting from state $k \in \{0, \dots, m\}$, the chain $\{Y(n)\}_{n \ge 0}$ hits m before it is absorbed at 0 is given by

$$\pi_k = \frac{1 - r^k}{1 - r^m}.$$

This is a classical result, which is the solution of the so-called gambler's ruin problem. To establish this, note that necessarily,

$$\pi_0 = 0, \; \pi_m = 1, \; (1 + r)\pi_k = r\pi_{k+1} + \pi_{k-1}, \; k \in \{1, \ldots, m - 1\}, \qquad (8.16)$$

and verify that the only solution to these relations is the one given above.

Thus, the probability that process $\{Z(t)\}_{t \geq 0}$ pays at least s visits to state m before being absorbed at 0 is the probability that the chain $\{Y(n)\}_{n \geq 0}$ pays at least s visits to state m. By (8.16), this reads

$$\mathbf{P}(\{Y(n)\}_{n \geq 0} \text{ visits state } m \text{ at least } s \text{ times}) = \frac{1 - r}{1 - r^m} \left(\frac{1 - r^{m-1}}{1 - r^m} \right)^s.$$

After each entrance into state m, process $\{Z(t)\}_{t \geq 0}$ remains there for an exponentially distributed sojourn time, with mean $1/m$. Thus, the probability that process $\{Z(t)\}_{t \geq 0}$ is not absorbed by time $s/2m$ satisfies

$$\mathbf{P}(Z(s/2m) > 0) \geq \mathbf{P}\left(\sum_{i=1}^{s} E_i \geq s/2 \right) \frac{1 - r}{1 - r^m} \left(\frac{1 - r^{m-1}}{1 - r^m} \right)^s,$$

where the random variables E_i are i.i.d., exponentially distributed with mean 1. Chernoff's Lemma 1.8 implies that the first term on the right-hand side satisfies

$$\mathbf{P}\left(\sum_{i=1}^{s} E_i \geq s/2 \right) \geq 1 - \exp\left(-s h_{\exp}(1/2) \right),$$

where

$$\begin{aligned} h_{\exp}(x) &= \sup_{\theta \in \mathbb{R}} \left(\theta x - \log \mathbf{E}(\exp(\theta E_1)) \right) \\ &= \sup_{\theta \in \mathbb{R}} \left(\theta x - \log(1/(1 - \theta)) \right) \\ &= x - 1 - \log x. \end{aligned}$$

The term $\exp(-s h_{\exp}(1/2))$ is clearly $o(s^{-1})$, and the result (8.14) follows. $\quad\square$

The main application of this result is captured in the following corollary.

Corollary 8.9 *Consider a sequence of finite graphs G_n on n nodes, a base infection rate β_n and an integer $m_n \geq n^a$, where a is a fixed positive constant, such that*

$$\beta_n \eta(m_n, G_n) \geq \frac{1}{r}, \qquad (8.17)$$

where $r \in (0, 1)$ is fixed. Then, denoting by τ_n the time to extinction of the contact process on G_n, with parameter β_n, it holds that

$$\mathbf{E}(\tau_n) \geq \exp(b n^a), \qquad (8.18)$$

for some positive constant $b > 0$.

Proof Let $n > 0$ be fixed. By (8.14), it holds that for all $s \in \mathbb{N}$,

$$\mathbf{E}(\tau_n) \geq \frac{s}{2m} \frac{1-r}{1-r^m} \left(\frac{1-r^{m-1}}{1-r^m} \right)^s \left(1 - o(s^{-1})\right),$$

where $m = m_n$. Take now $s = \lfloor r^{-m+1} \rfloor$ in the above expression to obtain

$$
\begin{aligned}
\mathbf{E}(\tau_n) \quad & \geq \frac{\lfloor r^{-m+1} \rfloor}{2m} \frac{1-r}{1-r^m} \left(\frac{1-r^{m-1}}{1-r^m} \right)^s \left(1 - o(s^{-1})\right) \\
& \geq (1-r)(1 - O(r^m))^{\frac{\lfloor r^{-m+1} \rfloor}{2m}} \left(1 - r^{m-1} \frac{1-r}{1-r^m}\right)^{r^{-m+1}} \\
& \geq (1-r)(1 - O(r^m))^{\frac{\lfloor r^{-m+1} \rfloor}{2m}} \exp(-(1-r)/(1-r^m)) \\
& \geq \frac{1-r}{e}(1 - O(r^m)) \exp(\log(1/r)(m-1) - \log 2m).
\end{aligned}
$$

For $m \geq n^a$, the exponent $\log(1/r)(m-1) - \log(2m)$ is clearly larger than bn^a for some suitable constant $b > 0$ (taking e.g. $b = \log(1/r)/2)$, and the result follows. $\qquad \square$

8.4 Epidemics on specific graphs

8.4.1 Application to hypercubes

The hypercube is a typical example of a logical topology used in so-called *distributed hash tables* (or DHTs). These provide a basic routing functionality. Namely, given one node of the graph and the address of a destination node, simple distributed algorithms enable a message to reach the destination in a small (logarithmic in the graph size) number of hops.

Here we represent a hypercube as a graph G with node set $\{0, 1\}^\ell$ for some $\ell \in \mathbb{N}$, and where the edge (v, w) is present if and only if the Hamming distance $d_H(v, w)$ equals 1.[2]

Because a hypercube is a regular graph, its spectral radius is $\rho = \log_2 n = \ell$. Hence, we have by Theorem 8.1 and Corollary 8.6:

- *Reed–Frost model*: If $\beta \log_2 n < 1 - c$, for some constant $c > 0$, then the expected final size of the epidemic is bounded by c times the number of initial infectives.

- *SIS model*: If $\beta \log_2 n < 1 - c$ for some constant $c > 0$, the epidemic dies out quickly (in time logarithmic in n). Let us now apply Corollary 8.9, to determine a condition under which the SIS epidemic dies out slowly. To this end, we will apply the following result established by Harper [39].

---

[2] For two words $v = v_1 \cdots v_\ell$ and $w = w_1 \cdots w_\ell$, the *Hamming distance* between v and w is $d_H(v, w) = \sum_{i=1}^\ell \delta_{v_i, w_i}$, where δ is the Kronecker symbol ($\delta_{ij} = 1$ if $i = j$, $\delta_{ij} = 0$ if $i \neq j$).

Lemma 8.10 *Let S be a set of m nodes of the hypercube $\{0,1\}^{\ell}$. Then $E(S,\bar{S})$ is larger than $E(S^*,\bar{S}^*)$, where S^* denotes the set of m smallest nodes according to the lexicographic order.*

For $k \le \ell$, we take $m = 2^k$. By Lemma 8.10, the set S^* realising the minimum isoperimetric ratio is the one comprising nodes $0^{l-j+1}x_1^{j-1}$, where x_1^{j-1} spans the whole set $\{0,1\}^{j-1}$, plus some points of type $0^{l-j}1x_1^{j-1}$, for some $j \le k$. Note that any point $y_1^{l-j}z_1^j$ with a unique 1 in the coordinates of y_1^{l-j} and such that $0^{l-j}z_1^j$ belongs to S^*, contributes exactly one edge to $E(S^*,\bar{S}^*)$. This yields the lower bound

$$E(S^*,\bar{S}^*) \ge (\ell - j)|S^*| \,.$$

From this one deduces that for $m = 2^k$, $\eta(m) \ge (\ell - k)$. In turn this yields the lower bound

$$\eta(m) \ge \log_2 n - \lceil \log_2 m \rceil, \quad m \in \{1,\dots,m\}. \tag{8.19}$$

Assume that, for some constant $c > 0$, one has

$$\beta \log_2 n > \frac{1}{1-c} \,.$$

One can then find another constant $\epsilon > 0$ (take e.g. $\epsilon = c/2$) such that

$$\beta(1 - \epsilon)\log_2 n > \frac{1}{1 - \epsilon} \,.$$

This, together with (8.19), implies that (8.17) holds with $m = \lfloor n^{\epsilon} \rfloor$ and $r = 1 - \epsilon$. The epidemics then last on average for time of order $\exp(bn^{\epsilon})$.

Thus for the hypercube, the behaviour of the SIS epidemics undergoes a sharp transition as the product $\beta \log_2 n$ crosses the critical value 1.

8.4.2 Application to star networks

The star-shaped network is of interest because it illustrates that the bounds in Theorem 8.1 and Corollary 8.6 are close to the best possible for general networks. It also exhibits a smooth dependence of the final size of the epidemic on the infectiousness parameter β, thereby demonstrating that threshold behaviour does not always occur. Finally, understanding the star is important to understanding certain power-law networks.

Consider the star network consisting of a hub and $n-1$ leaves, each of which is attached only to the hub. Its adjacency matrix A has ones along the first row and column, except for the $(1, 1)$ element, which is zero; all other elements are zero. Thus A is a rank-two matrix and can have only two non-zero eigenvalues. It is readily verified that $(\sqrt{n-1}, 1, \ldots, 1)^T$ and $(-\sqrt{n-1}, 1, \ldots, 1)^T$ are eigenvectors corresponding to the eigenvalues $\sqrt{n-1}$ and $-\sqrt{n-1}$ respectively, and so the spectral radius of A is $\sqrt{n-1}$.

- *Reed–Frost model*: Suppose that $\beta\sqrt{n-1} = c < 1$. Consider the initial condition where only the hub is infected, so that $|X(0)| = 1$. The number of leaves infected before the hub is cured is binomial with parameters $n-1$ and β. No other leaves can be infected subsequently. Hence,

$$\mathbf{E}\left[|Y(\infty)|\right] = 1 + \beta(n-1) = 1 + c\sqrt{n-1},$$

which is comparable to the upper bound, $\sqrt{n-1}/(1-c)$, given by Theorem 8.1. In addition, Chernoff's inequality (see Lemma 1.8) implies that, for $c' < c$, $\mathbf{P}\left(|Y(\infty)| < c'\sqrt{n}\right)$ goes to 0, exponentially in n, when n goes to infinity.

We observe in this case that $\mathbf{E}\left[|Y(\infty)|\right]$ is a smooth (almost linear) function of β and does not exhibit any threshold behaviour.

Suppose next that the hub is initially uninfected but k leaves are infected. The hub becomes infected at the next time step with probability $1-(1-\beta)^k$. It subsequently infects a number of leaves which is binomial with parameters $n-1-k$ and β. The epidemic dies out at $t = 3$. So, in this case,

$$\mathbf{E}\left[|Y(\infty)|\right] = k + [1 - (1-\beta)^k][1 + \beta(n-1-k)]$$
$$\leq k + \beta k[1 + \beta(n-1-k)] \leq |X(0)|(1 + 2c^2).$$

Thus, when the hub is initially uninfected, the expected final size of the epidemic is only a constant multiple of the initial number of infectives. This illustrates that the initial condition can have a big impact in general.

- *SIS model*: In the case of the SIS model, it is not difficult to see that the isoperimetric constant is equal to 1. Hence, the application of Corollaries 8.6 and 8.9 to the star-shaped network implies that (i) the epidemic dies out quickly provided that $\beta < 1/\sqrt{n}$, and (ii) it dies out slowly provided that $\beta > 1$. These results are loose; tighter thresholds can be derived by performing a detailed study of the epidemics on this topology (see [36]).

8.4.3 Application to complete graphs

A complete graph is one in which an edge is present between every pair of nodes. Much of the early work on SIR epidemics was based on mean-field models. These are rigorously justifiable only in the case of complete graphs, and this motivates our interest in such graphs.

We shall recover the classical result that the epidemic has a threshold at $R_0 = 1$, where the basic reproduction number $R_0 = \beta(n - 1)$ is defined as the mean number of secondary infections caused by a single primary infective, when the entire population is susceptible.

- *Reed–Frost model*: The complete graph is a regular graph with common node degree $n - 1$. Therefore, its spectral radius is $\rho = n - 1$, and we have by Theorem 8.1 that, if $\beta(n - 1) < 1$, then the final size of the epidemic is bounded by $1/(1 - \beta(n - 1))$ times the initial number of infectives. We now establish a converse.

Suppose $\beta(n - 1) = c > 1$ is held constant. Let $|X_0| = 1$ and let u be the initial infected node. Consider the random subgraph of the complete graph obtained by retaining each edge with probability β, independent of all other edges, and let $C(u)$ denote the connected component containing u in this random graph (possibly just the singleton $\{u\}$).

As already discussed in Chapter 2, it is clear that $C(u)$ can be interpreted as the set of infected nodes in the epidemic. Thus, the number of infected nodes in the epidemic has the same probability law as the size of the component $C(u)$.

This random graph model was introduced by Erdős and Rényi [30]; we denote it by $G(n,\beta)$, where n is the number of nodes, and β the probability that the edge between each pair of nodes is present.

We now use the following fact, presented in Chapter 2, which was first established by Erdős and Rényi [30]; see [42, theorem 5.4] for a more recent reference. Here, we assume that $c = \beta(n - 1)$ is held constant while $n \to \infty$, and that $c > 1$.

Theorem 8.11 *Let γ be the unique positive solution of $\gamma + e^{-\gamma c} = 1$. Then, as $n \to \infty$, the size of the largest connected component in the random graph $G(n,\beta)$ is $(1 + o(1))\gamma n$, with probability going to 1 as n tends to infinity.*

We now estimate the size of $C(u)$, the connected component containing the initial infective. If u belongs to the 'giant component', then $|C(u)| = (1 + o(1))\gamma n$. Since a fraction γ of nodes belong to the giant component, the probability that node u does so is γ. Hence, $\mathbf{E}\left[|C(u)|\right] = (1 + o(1))\gamma^2 n$. Moreover, it is proved in Theorem 2.1 that the size of the second largest component in the supercritical random graph is $O(\log n)$. Hence $|Y(\infty)| = O(\log n)$ with probability $1 - \gamma$, which is the probability that the initial node does not belong to the giant component, and $\mathbf{P}(|Y(\infty)| > (1 + o(1))\gamma n) = \gamma$. We have thus shown the following.

Theorem 8.12   *Let G = (V, E) be the complete graph on n nodes, and let $\beta = \frac{c}{n-1}$ for an arbitrary constant c > 1. Then, the final size of the epidemic satisfies*

$$\mathbf{E}\left[|Y(\infty)|\right] \geq (1 + o(1))\gamma^2 n,$$

for any $|X(0)| \geq 1$, where $\gamma > 0$ solves $\gamma + e^{-\gamma c} = 1$. Moreover, $|Y(\infty)| = O(\log n)$ with probability $1 - \gamma$.

There is thus a threshold at $c = 1$ for the final size of the epidemic; starting with a constant number of initial infectives, the final size is a constant independent of n if $c < 1$, and a fraction of n if $c > 1$.

- *SIS model*: The isoperimetric constant $\eta(m)$ is easily shown to be $n - m$. Applying Corollaries 8.6 and 8.9 tells us that the epidemic dies out quickly when $\beta < 1/(n - 1)$ and slowly when $\beta > 1/(n - m)$, where $m = n^a$ for some $a > 0$. Thus $1/n$ is essentially the correct threshold and, as in the case of the hypercube, there is no gap.

8.4.4 Application to E-R graphs

The Erdős-Rényi graph $G(n, p)$ with parameters n and p is defined as a random graph on n nodes, where the edge between each pair of nodes is present with probability p, independent of all other edges.

Let $d := (n - 1)p$ denote the expected degree of an arbitrary node. We consider the regime $\log n \ll d$, i.e. $\log(n)/d \to 0$ as $n \to \infty$.

- *Reed–Frost model*: Consider a sequence of such graphs indexed by n. Define $c_n = \beta d = (n - 1)\beta p$; we have suppressed the dependence of β and p on n in the notation, but make it explicit in the case of c. Consider an SIR epidemic on such a graph starting with one node initially infected. We have the following.

Theorem 8.13   *If $\limsup_{n\to\infty} c_n \leq c < 1$, then for all n sufficiently large, $\mathbf{E}\left[|Y(\infty)|\right]$ is bounded by a constant that does not depend on n.*

   On the other hand, if $\liminf_{n\to\infty} c_n \geq c > 1$, then $\mathbf{E}\left[|Y(\infty)|\right] \geq (1 + o(1))\gamma^2 n$ and $|Y(\infty)| = O(\log n)$ with probability $1 - \gamma$ where $\gamma > 0$ solves $\gamma + e^{-\gamma c} = 1$.

Proof   Suppose first that $\liminf_{n\to\infty} c_n \geq c > 1$. As in the case of the complete graph, we identify the infected individuals in the epidemic with the connected component containing the initial infective u in an Erdős-Rényi random graph with parameters n and βp. (If edge (u, v) is present in the original Erdős-Rényi graph, which happens with probability p, then u succeeds in infecting v with probability p. This yields the new graph with edge probability βp; the independence of the edges is obvious.) Thus, the second claim of the theorem follows in the same way as Theorem 8.12.

The first claim is stronger than what the upper bound of Theorem 8.1 yields. Note that, by the Perron–Frobenius theorem, the spectral radius ρ of the adjacency matrix lies between the smallest and largest node degrees. For the random graph $G(n, p)$, the node degrees are binomial random variables with parameters $n-1$ and p. If the average node degree $d = (n-1)p$ satisfies $d \gg \log n$, i.e. $(\log n)/d \to 0$ as $n \to \infty$, then it can be shown using the Chernoff bound that both the minimal and maximal node degrees are $(1 + o(1))d$ with high probability; hence, so is the spectral radius. In this case, Theorem 8.1 yields that, if $\beta\rho \sim (n-1)\beta p \leq c < 1$, then the expected final size of the epidemic is bounded by a constant times $\sqrt{n}$. To show that it is in fact bounded by a constant, and that this holds even without the assumption that $d \gg \log n$, we use a branching process construction.

Rather than fixing the random graph $G(n, p)$ in advance, we use the principle of deferred decisions to generate it dynamically as the epidemic progresses. Thus, starting with the initial infective u, we put down all edges from u to other nodes. Then, we decide whether u succeeds in infecting its neighbours along each of those edges. For each neighbour v so infected, we repeat the process.

Thus, the number of nodes infected by u is binomial with parameters $n - 1$ and βp; the number of nodes infected by each subsequent infective is stochastically dominated by such a binomial random variable. Thus, the size of the epidemic is bounded above by the size of a branching process whose offspring distribution is binomial, $\text{Bin}(n - 1, \beta p)$. The branching process is subcritical by the assumption that $(n - 1)\beta p \leq c < 1$, and so it becomes extinct with probability 1, i.e., its final population size is finite almost surely.

It turns out that the final population size is also finite, and uniformly bounded in n. This follows easily from Theorem 1.2. □

- *SIS model*: We first derive the asymptotic behaviour of the isoperimetric constant η when n goes to infinity.

Theorem 8.14 *Let m be such that $m/n \to \alpha$ as $n \to \infty$, for a fixed $\alpha \in (0, 1)$. Assume further that $\log n \ll d$. Then it holds that, with high probability,*

$$\eta(G, m) = (1 + o(1))(1 - \alpha)d. \tag{8.20}$$

Proof Fix some $k \in (0, 1 - \alpha)$. By the union bound,

$$\mathbf{P}(\eta(G, m) < kd) \le \sum_{i=1}^{m} \sum_{S:|S|=i} \mathbf{P}\left(E(S, \overline{S}) < kdi\right).$$

Note that $E(S, \overline{S})$ has a binomial distribution with parameters $i(n - i)$ and p. Denote by $\mathrm{Bin}(i(n - i), p)$ a generic binomial random variable with this distribution. We thus have

$$\mathbf{P}(\eta(G, m) < kd) \le \sum_{i=1}^{m} \binom{n}{i} \mathbf{P}\left(\mathrm{Bin}(i(n - i), p) < kdi\right).$$

Since $k < 1 - \alpha$ and $m = (1 + o(1))\alpha n$, we have for n large enough that $(n - i)p > kd$ for all $i \in \{1, \ldots, m\}$ and that $(n - 1)/(n - i) \le 1/(1 - \alpha)$. We now apply the Chernoff bound

$$P\left(B < (1 - \delta)\mathbf{E}(B)\right) < e^{-\mathbf{E}(B)\delta^2/2}, \tag{8.21}$$

valid for any binomial random variable B, to $\mathrm{Bin}(i(n - i), p)$ in the above expression. Taking

$$\delta = 1 - k\frac{n - 1}{n - i} \ge 1 - \frac{k}{1 - \alpha},$$

this yields

$$\mathbf{P}\left(\eta(G, m) < kd\right) \le \sum_{i=1}^{m} \binom{n}{i} e^{-i(n-i)p\epsilon}, \tag{8.22}$$

where $\epsilon = \frac{1}{2}\left(1 - \frac{k}{1-\alpha}\right)^2 > 0$. We thus have the upper bound

$$\mathbf{P}(\eta(G, m) < kd) \le \sum_{i=1}^{m} \frac{n^i}{i!} e^{-i(n-i)p\epsilon}$$

$$= \sum_{i=1}^{m} \frac{1}{i!} e^{-i((n-i)p\epsilon - \log n)},$$

where we have also used the upper bound $\binom{n}{i} \le n^i/i!$ to obtain the first inequality. By assumption, $\log n \ll d = (n - 1)p$, and ϵ is a positive constant that does not depend on n. Thus, for any constant $K > 0$, it holds that, for n large enough,

$$\mathbf{P}\left(\eta(G, m) < kd\right) \le \sum_{i=1}^{m} \frac{1}{i!} n^{-Ki} \le \exp\left(n^{-K}\right) - 1.$$

This suffices to conclude that for any $k < 1 - \alpha$, with high probability $\eta(G, m) \ge kd$.

In order to obtain an inequality in the opposite direction, choose any set S of cardinality m. Then one has

$$\eta(G, m) \leq \frac{E(S, \overline{S})}{m} .$$

Let $k > (1 - \alpha)$ be fixed. One then has

$$\mathbf{P}(\eta(G, m) > kd) \leq \mathbf{P}(\text{Bin}(m(n - m), p) > km(n - 1)p) .$$

It is readily seen using a Chernoff bound that the right-hand side goes to zero as $n \rightarrow \infty$. This concludes the proof of the theorem. $\square$

Theorem 8.15 *Consider an Erdős–Rényi random graph $G(n, p)$ such that $\log n \ll d = np$. The following claims hold with high probability: an epidemic on $G(n, p)$ dies out quickly, $E[\tau] = O(\log n)$, provided $\beta < (1-u)/d$ for $0 < u < 1$. On the other hand, the epidemic dies out slowly, $\log E[\tau] = \Omega(n)$ provided that $\beta > (1 + v)/d$ for $v > 0$.*

Proof The theorem follows from Corollaries 8.6 and 8.9, the expression $\rho(A) = (1 + o(1))d$ for the spectral radius, and Theorem 8.14. $\square$

Thus as for the hypercube and the complete graph, there is a sharp transition in the behaviour of SIS epidemics on Erdős–Rényi graphs in the regime $d \gg \log n$ as the product βd crosses the critical value 1.

8.5 Notes

The material in this chapter is adapted from the articles by Draief, Massoulié, Ganesh, Towsley [36, 27]. In these papers the authors apply the above results to other families of graphs of interest, among which are power-law networks.

More recently, Britton, Janson and Martin-Löf considered the Reed–Frost model on a random graph with a prespecified degree distribution that accounts for the social structure in a large community [17]. They determine the basic reproduction number, the asymptotic final size and the impact of local vaccination strategies in the case of a major outbreak.

9

Viral marketing and optimised epidemics

9.1 Model and motivation

In Chapter 8 we tried to understand the impact of a network's topology on the behaviour of epidemics. In the present chapter, we focus on the role played by the initial condition in determining the size of the epidemic. Moreover, we adopt a different viewpoint, taking an algorithmic perspective. That is to say, we address the following question: given a set of individuals that form a network, how should one choose a subset of these individuals, of given size, to be infected initially, so as to maximise the size of an epidemic? The idea is that by carefully choosing such nodes we could trigger a cascade of infections that will result in a large number of ultimately infected individuals.

This problem finds its motivation in viral marketing. In this context, limited advertising budget is available for the purpose of convincing a small number of consumers (i.e. the size of the set of initial infectives) of the merits of some product. Such consumers may in turn convince others, and the aim is to maximise the ultimate reach of the advertisement by leveraging such "contaminations".

We address this problem by considering the following version of the Reed–Frost epidemic. We assume that the network is described by a directed graph G. The potentially infected individuals constitute the set $V := \{1, \ldots, n\}$. For each ordered pair of individuals $(i, j) \in V \times V$, the probability that i, if infected, will contaminate j is denoted p_{ij}. The occurrences of such infection propagations are assumed independent across all pairs (i, j).

Let C denote the set of initially infected nodes. Let $U(C)$ denote the corresponding set of ultimately infected nodes. Then $U(C)$ can be characterised as the set of nodes in V that can be reached from C by a directed path of edges in graph G. Eventually, we address the following problem. Given weights p_{ij} as above, and some "infection budget" $k < n$, identify the set C of size k that maximises the expected outbreak size, $\mathbf{E}\,(|U(C)|)$. For notational convenience, we shall denote it by $F(C)$:

$$F(C) := \mathbf{E}\,(|U(C)|)\,.$$

We shall first show that this problem is algorithmically hard, then identify a particular structure underlying the problem, namely submodularity. We shall provide generic results on the performance of a "greedy" procedure for the maximisation of a submodular function, and finally apply these results to show how greedy approaches combined with statistical sampling yield efficient solutions to the problem of maximising outbreak size.

9.2 Algorithmic hardness

Let us show that this generic problem is hard to solve. To this end, we use a *reduction* argument, whereby an efficient procedure to solve the above problem can be turned into an efficient procedure to solve the so-called *set-cover* problem [75], to be described shortly. Since the set-cover problem is *NP-hard*, we deduce as a result that no polynomial-time procedure exists for solving the outbreak maximisation problem, unless the celebrated conjecture "P≠NP" is false.

In the set-cover problem, one is given a finite set C_0 and a collection $C_1, \ldots,$ C_m of m nonempty subsets of C_0. The problem then consists of determining whether there exist k such subsets, the union of which is exactly C_0.

Given such an instance of the set-cover problem, consider the following instance of epidemic outbreak maximisation. The node set V is chosen as the union of $\{1, \ldots, m\}$ with C_0, assuming the two sets are disjoint. The probability p_{ij} is then chosen as 1 if $i \in \{1, \ldots, m\}$ and $j \in C_i$, and zero otherwise. It is readily seen that for any set C of initially infected nodes satisfying $|C| = k$ and $C \subset \{1, \ldots, m\}$ the size $|U(C)|$ equals $k + |\cup_{i \in C} C_i|$. In addition, only sets satisfying these conditions need to be considered to maximise the ultimate outbreak.

Thus, there exists a set C of size k leading to an ultimate outbreak of size $|U(C)| = k + |C_0|$ if and only if the set-cover problem admits a solution. Therefore, an algorithm returning an optimal initial set C can be turned into an algorithm for deciding feasibility of the set-cover problem. Furthermore, the artificial outbreak maximisation problem constructed above takes as input a node set of size $m + |C_0|$, together with $\{0, 1\}$-valued infection probabilities p_{ij}. This input size is polynomial in the size of the input specification of the considered set-cover problem. This establishes the desired reduction property.

9.3 Submodular structure and its consequences

In this section we analyse the properties of the influence function F that to a subset C of initially infected nodes associates $F(C) = \mathbf{E}(|U(C)|)$, the average size of the set of ultimately infected nodes.

The marketer's objective is to choose a subset C that maximises $F(C)$. As shown in Section 9.2, this problem is NP-hard, so the best the marketer can achieve is to approximate the optimal value. Although it is not the case for a general influence model as discussed in [48], the model we are interested in falls within a subclass of models for which one can obtain good approximation results.

This subclass corresponds to models where the influence function is monotone and submodular. Monotonicity ensures that the larger the size of the initial set of infectives, the more nodes are infected ultimately. Submodularity corresponds to the phenomenon of diminishing returns whereby, beyond a certain size of the set of initial infectives C, the marginal effect of adding more nodes to C decreases. More precisely:

Definition 9.1 (Submodularity)   A real-valued function F, defined on the set of subsets C of some basic set V, is *submodular* if for all $A, B \subseteq V$, the following inequality holds:

$$F(A \cup B) + F(A \cap B) \leq F(A) + F(B) . \tag{9.1}$$

Given some directed graph $G = (V, E)$, let us denote as before by $U(C)$ the set of nodes j that can be reached from some node $i \in C$ via a directed path of edges in E. Then the function $C \to |U(C)|$ is submodular. Indeed, it is easily shown that

$$U(A \cup B) = U(A) \cup U(B) ,$$

so that

$$|U(A \cup B)| = |U(A)| + |U(B)| - |U(A) \cap U(B)| .$$

However, the set-valued function $C \to U(C)$ is clearly non-decreasing, so that $U(A \cap B) \subset U(A)$ and $U(A \cap B) \subset U(B)$. Hence, $U(A \cap B) \subset U(A) \cap U(B)$. Combined with the previous displayed equation, this yields

$$|U(A \cup B)| + |U(A \cap B)|$$
$$= |U(A)| + |U(B)| - |U(A) \cap U(B)| + |U(A \cap B)| \leq |U(A)| + |U(B)| ,$$

which is precisely the definition of submodularity.

Consequently, the influence function in the outbreak maximisation problem, which reads $F(C) := \mathbf{E}(|U(C)|)$, is also submodular. Indeed, a random function that is submodular with probability 1 is such that its expectation is also submodular: this follows by taking expectations in the defining inequality (9.1).

Given some function F over subsets C of some basic set V, a naive method of identifying a subset C of target size k with large corresponding value $F(C)$ consists on the following *greedy procedure*. Choose items $v_1, \ldots, v_k \in V$ recursively as follows:

$$v_i \in \text{argmax}_{v \in V \setminus C_{i-1}}\{F(C_{i-1} \cup \{v\})\}, \quad i = 1, \ldots, k,$$

where $C_0 = \emptyset$ and $C_j = \{v_1, \ldots, v_j\}$, $j = 1, \ldots, k - 1$. Then set $C = C_k$. It will be useful to consider a relaxed requirement for iterative selection of the v_i. Given some fixed constant $\epsilon \in (0, 1]$ and $\delta \geq 0$, we shall say that the sequence $v_1, \ldots, v_k$ is (ϵ, δ)-greedy if it satisfies the following inequalities:

$$F(C_{i-1} \cup \{v_i\}) - F(C_{i-1})$$
$$\geq \epsilon \max_{v \in V \setminus C_{i-1}} (F(C_{i-1} \cup \{v\}) - F(C_{i-1})) - \delta, \ i = 1, \ldots, k. \quad (9.2)$$

Thus, a $(1,0)$-greedy sequence is exactly a greedy sequence according to the previous definition.

The submodular structure has an important consequence.

Theorem 9.2 *Consider a function $F : 2^V \to \mathbb{R}$ that takes non-negative values, is submodular and is non-decreasing in the sense that $F(C) \leq F(D)$ if $C \subset D$. Let $v_1, \ldots, v_k$ be an (ϵ, δ)-greedy sequence of elements of V. Then the following holds:*

$$F(C_k) \geq (1 - e^{-\epsilon}) \max_{C \subset V, |C| = k} F(C) - \frac{k\delta}{\epsilon}. \quad (9.3)$$

That is to say, an (ϵ, δ)-greedy sequential selection of elements identifies a set C_k with value at least $(1 - e^{-\epsilon})$ times the maximum value that can be achieved by arbitrary sets C of size k, minus some absolute difference no larger than $k\delta/\epsilon$.

Proof Let some subset $C = \{w_1, \ldots, w_k\}$ of V, of size k, be fixed. For an arbitrary index $i \in \{1, \ldots, k - 1\}$, we claim that

$$F(C_{i+1}) - F(C_i) \geq \frac{\epsilon}{k} [F(C) - F(C_i)] - \delta, \quad (9.4)$$

where C_i is the set $\{v_1, \ldots, v_i\}$ of the i first elements in an arbitrary (ϵ, δ)-greedy sequence. To establish (9.4), we proceed as follows. For all $j = 0, \ldots, k$, define the set D_j as

$$D_j = C_i \cup \{w_1, \ldots, w_j\},$$

so that $D_0 = C_i$ and $D_k = C_i \cup C$. Thus

$$\sum_{j=1}^{k} F(D_j) - F(D_{j-1}) = F(C_i \cup C) - F(C_i) \geq F(C) - F(C_i),$$

by monotonicity of F. Therefore there must exist $j \in \{1, \ldots, k\}$ such that

$$F(D_j) - F(D_{j-1}) \geq \frac{1}{k} [F(C) - F(C_i)]. \tag{9.5}$$

Now submodularity of F implies that

$$F(C_i \cup \{w_j\}) + F(D_{j-1}) \geq F(C_i) + F(D_j),$$

or equivalently

$$F(C_i \cup \{w_j\}) - F(C_i) \geq F(D_j) - F(D_{j-1}).$$

This combined with (9.5) yields

$$F(C_i \cup \{w_j\}) - F(C_i) \geq \frac{1}{k} [F(C) - F(C_i)].$$

By definition of an (ϵ, δ)-greedy sequence, the left-hand side of (9.4) is at least ϵ times the left-hand side of the last inequality, minus δ; (9.4) then follows.

A direct consequence is

$$F(C) - F(C_{i+1}) \leq \left(1 - \frac{\epsilon}{k}\right)[F(C) - F(C_i)] + \delta.$$

By induction, this last inequality yields

$$F(C) - F(C_k)$$

$$\leq \left(1 - \frac{\epsilon}{k}\right)^k [F(C) - F(C_0)] + \delta \sum_{i=0}^{k-1} \left(1 - \frac{\epsilon}{k}\right)^i \leq \left(1 - \frac{\epsilon}{k}\right)^k F(C) + \frac{k\delta}{\epsilon}.$$

Noting that

$$\left(1 - \frac{\epsilon}{k}\right)^k \leq e^{-\epsilon},$$

the result (9.3) follows.   □

9.4 Viral marketing

The idea of using viral marketing as a means of diffusing new trends, behaviours and innovations through social networks has attracted growing interest from the social science community [78, 80]. Driven by the recent growth of the Internet, computer scientists have joined this endeavour, motivated by phenomena such as information propagation through blogs [38], recommendation systems [56] and other applications of Web 2.0.

Driven by the belief that consumers' purchasing decisions are strongly influenced by referrals from their neighbours in a social network, a number of techniques have been developed to analyse diffusion properties in large-scale social networks. As an example of viral marketing, consider a company that wishes to promote its new instant messenger (IM) system [61]. A promising way would be through a popular social network such as MySpace: by convincing several people to adopt the new IM system, the company can initiate an effective marketing campaign and diffuse the new system over the network. To find an effective set of initial adopters C, the company would need to estimate the influence function $F(C)$ for the network.

In this section we address the question of estimating $F(C)$ based on the knowledge about the social network of interest, MySpace in our example. To this end, we explain how to apply Theorem 9.2 to viral marketing. One difficulty arises because the function F, representing the expected number of infectives, is characterised by the infection probabilities p_{ij}. No computationally efficient procedure is known for computing $F(C)$ exactly from these probabilities. We therefore resort to simulation methods.

More precisely, when we set out to estimate $F(C)$ for some particular set C, we generate M i.i.d. samples of random graphs, denoted $G_1, \ldots, G_M$, corresponding to the edge probabilities p_{ij}. We then estimate $F(C)$ by $\hat{F}(C)$, i.e. the empirical average of the M sampled values, denoted $U_1(C), \ldots, U_M(C)$. Since the underlying random variables $U_i(C)$ are $\{0, \ldots, n\}$-valued, where $n = |V|$, an application of the Chernoff bound implies that for all $\gamma > 0$,

$$\mathbf{P}\left(|\hat{F}(C) - F(C)| \geq \gamma F(C)\right) \leq 2e^{-Mh(\gamma/n)} ,$$

where h denotes the Cramér transform of a centred unit-mean Poisson random variable, i.e.

$$h(x) := (1 + x)\log(1 + x) - x .$$

Let us determine the relative precision δ such that, if the estimates $\hat{F}(C)$ satisfy $|\hat{F}(C) - F(C)| \leq \gamma F(C)$, a greedy construction of a sequence $v_1, \ldots, v_k$ based on the estimates $\hat{F}(C_i \cup \{v\})$ is necessarily an (ϵ, δ)-greedy sequence, according to the definition given in (9.2). The sequence $v_1, \ldots, v_k$ is chosen so that

$$\hat{F}(C_{i+1}) - \hat{F}(C_i) = \max_{v \in V}\left\{\hat{F}(C_i \cup \{v\}) - \hat{F}(C_i)\right\} .$$

Provided the estimates $\hat{F}$ have relative error at most γ, then

$$\frac{1}{1 - \gamma} F(C_{i+1}) - \frac{1}{1 + \gamma} F(C_i) \geq \max_{v \in V} \left\{ \frac{1}{1 + \gamma} F(C_i \cup \{v\}) - \frac{1}{1 - \gamma} F(C_i) \right\} .$$

Elementary manipulations lead to

$$\frac{F(C_{i+1}) - F(C_i)}{1 - \gamma} + \frac{2\gamma}{1 - \gamma^2} F(C_i)$$

$$\geq \max_{v \in V} \left[\frac{F(C_i \cup \{v\}) - F(C_i)}{1 + \gamma} - \frac{2\gamma}{1 - \gamma^2} F(C_i \cup \{v\}) \right] .$$

Since the function F is bounded by n, eventually this shows that the constructed sequence is (ϵ, δ)-greedy, with

$$\epsilon = \frac{1 - \gamma}{1 + \gamma}, \quad \delta = \frac{4\gamma n}{1 + \gamma} . \tag{9.6}$$

We are now in a position to prove the following result.

Proposition 9.3 *Let $r > 0$ be a fixed number. Assume that M random graphs are generated at each step of the greedy construction procedure, to form the estimates $\hat{F}(C_i \cup \{v\})$ for all $v \in V \setminus C_i$ (hence, overall, kM random graphs). Then with probability at least*

$$1 - 2nke^{-Mh(r/n^2)} ,$$

the corresponding set C_k is such that

$$F(C_k) \geq (1 - e^{-1} - 4r - O(1/n)) \sup_{C \subset V, |C| = k} F(C) .$$

Proof By the previous argument and an application of Theorem 9.2, we have, setting $\gamma = r/n$, that with the desired probability,

$$F(C_k) \geq (1 - e^{-\epsilon}) \max_{C \subset V, |C| = k} F(C) - \frac{k\delta}{\epsilon} ,$$

where ϵ and δ are as in (9.6). Noting that for all C such that $|C| = k$, $F(C) \geq k$, we deduce that

$$F(C_k) \geq \left(1 - e^{-\epsilon} - \frac{\delta}{\epsilon} \right) \max_{C \subset V, |C| = k} F(C) .$$

Clearly, if we choose $\epsilon = 1 - O(1/n)$ and $\delta/\epsilon = 4r - O(1/n)$, then the result follows. □

Since $h(r/n^2) = \Theta(r^2/n^4)$,[1] it is readily seen that taking e.g. M of order $n^4 \log n$ is sufficient to ensure that $nke^{-Mh(r/n^2)} = o(1)$. Thus, for such M, with

---

[1] That is, there are $\delta_1, \delta_2 > 0$ such that $\delta_1(r^2/n^4) \leq h(r/n^2) \leq \delta_2(r^2/n^4)$.

high probability the proposed procedure identifies a set of nodes to be infected with a relative payoff of at least $(1 - e^{-1} - 4r - O(1/n))$ times the optimal value. That is to say, this probabilistic procedure enables us to determine with high probability, and polynomial complexity, a solution within a constant factor of the optimal, whereas determining the optimal is infeasible in polynomial time if $P \neq NP$.

9.5 Notes

The material in this chapter is adapted from the articles by Kempe, Kleinberg and Tardos [48, 44]. More general models of propagation are discussed in these articles, for which submodularity still holds. For the more general models, this submodularity property is conjectured in [44], and proven using clever coupling arguments in Mossel and Roch [70]. There have been a number of recent empirical investigations on diffusion in social networks, see [56, 49, 25].

The search for algorithms that provide guarantees on relative performance compared to an optimal solution, for NP-hard problems, is an active research topic, to which the book of Vazirani [81] is dedicated.

References

[1] D. Aldous, Brownian excursions, critical random graphs and the multiplicative coalescent, *Annals of Probability*, **25**(2), 812–854, 1997.

[2] N. Alon and J. H. Spencer, *The Probabilistic Method*, Wiley, New York, 2000.

[3] H. Andersson and T. Britton, *Stochastic Epidemic Models and Their Statistical Analysis*, Lecture Notes in Statistics, Springer, 2000.

[4] K. B. Athreya and P. E. Ney, *Branching Processes*, Dover, 2004.

[5] N. J. Bailey, *The Mathematical Theory of Epidemics*, Griffin, 1957.

[6] F. Ball, A threshold theorem for the Reed–Frost chain-binomial epidemic, *Journal of Applied Probability*, **20**(1), 153–157, 1983.

[7] F. Ball, D. Mollison and G. Scalia-Tomba, Epidemics with two levels of mixing, *Annals of Applied Probability*, **7**(1), 46–89, 1997.

[8] A.-L. Barabási and R. Albert, Emergence of scaling in random networks, *Science*, **286**, 509–512, 1999.

[9] A. D. Barbour, L. Holst, S. Janson and J. H. Spencer, *Poisson Approximations*, Oxford University Press, 1992.

[10] A. D. Barbour and D. Mollison, Epidemics and random graphs, in *Stochastic Processes in Epidemic Theory*, pp. 86–89. Lecture Notes in Biomathematics, 86, Springer, 1990.

[11] A. D. Barbour and S. Utev, Approximating the Reed–Frost epidemic process, *Stochastic Processes and Their Applications*, **113**, 173–197, 2004.

[12] K. P. Birman, M. Hayden, O. Ozkasap, Z. Xiao, M. Budiu and Y. Minsky, Bimodal multicast, *ACM Transactions on Computer Systems*, **17**(2), 41–88, 1999.

[13] B. Bollobás, *Random Graphs*, Cambridge University Press, 2nd edition, 2001.

[14] B. Bollobás, C. Borgs, J. T. Chayes and O. Riordan, Directed scale-free graphs, in *Proceedings of the Fourteenth ACM Symposium on Discrete Algorithms (SODA)*, pp. 132–139, 2003.

[15] B. Bollobás, S. Janson and O. Riordan, The phase transition in inhomogeneous random graphs, *Random Structures and Algorithms*, **31**(1), 3–122, 2007.

[16] B. Bollobás and O. Riordan, The diameter of a scale-free random graph, *Combinatorica*, **4**, 5–34, 2004.

[17] T. Britton, S. Janson and A. Martin-Löf, Graphs with specified degree distributions, simple epidemics, and local vaccination strategies, *Advances in Applied Probability*, **39**(4), 922–948, 2007.

[18] S. Chatterjee, P. Diaconis and E. Meckes, Exchangeable pairs and Poisson approximation, *Probability Surveys*, **2**, 64–106, 2005.

[19] F. Chung and L. Lu, Connected components in random graphs with given degree sequences, *Annals of Combinatorics*, **6**, 125–145, 2002.

[20] F. Chung and L. Lu, The average distances in random graphs with given expected degrees, *Internet Mathematics*, **1**, 91–114, 2003.

[21] F. Chung, L. Lu and V. Vu, Eigenvalues of random power law graphs, *Annals of Combinatorics*, **7**, 21–33, 2003.

[22] M. Costa, M. Castro, J. Crowcroft, A. Rowstron, L. Zhou, L. Zhang and P. Barham, Vigilante: end-to-end containment of Internet worms, in *Proceedings of the Twentieth ACM Symposium on Operating Systems Principles*, pp. 133–147, 2005.

[23] D. J. Daley and J. Gani, *Epidemic Modelling: An Introduction*, Cambridge University Press, 2001.

[24] P. Dodds and D. Watts, Universal behavior in a generalized model of contagion, *Physical Review Letters*, **92**, 218701, 2004.

[25] P. Domingos, Mining social networks for viral marketing, *IEEE Intelligent Systems*, **20**(1), 80–82, 2005.

[26] M. Draief and A. Ganesh, Efficient routing in Poisson small-world networks, *Journal of Applied Probability*, **43**, 678–686, 2006.

[27] M. Draief, A. Ganesh and L. Massoulié, Thresholds for virus spread on networks, *Annals of Applied Probability*, **18**(2), 359–378, 2008.

[28] R. Durrett, *Random Graph Dynamics*, Cambridge University Press, 2006.

[29] P. Erdős and A. Rényi, On random graphs I, *Publicationes Mathematicae Debrecen* **6**, 290–297, 1959.

[30] P. Erdős and A. Rényi, On the evolution of random graphs, *Publications of the Mathematical Institute of the Hungarian Academy of Science*, **5**, 17–61, 1960.

[31] P. Erdős and A. Rényi, On the evolution of random graphs, *Bulletin of the International Institute of Statistics Tokyo*, **38**, 343–347, 1961.

[32] S. N. Ethier and T. G. Kurtz, *Markov Processes: Characterization and Convergence*, Wiley, 1986.

[33] P. Eugster, R. Guerraoui, A.-M. Kermarrec and L. Massoulié, From epidemics to distributed computing, *IEEE Computer*, **37**(5), 60–67, 1999.

[34] M. Faloutsos, P. Faloutsos and C. Faloutsos, On power-law relationships of the Internet topology, in *Proceedings of the ACM Conference on Applications, Technologies, Architectures, and Protocols for Computer Communication (SIGCOMM)*, pp. 251–262, 1999.

[35] M. Franceschetti and R. Meester, *Random Networks for Communication: From Statistical Physics to Information Systems*, Cambridge University Press, 2008.

[36] A. Ganesh, L. Massoulié and D. Towsley, Effect of network topology on the spread of epidemics, in *Proceedings of the 24th Annual Joint Conference of the IEEE Computer and Communications Societies (INFOCOM)*, **2**, 1455–1466, 2005.

[37] A. Ganesh, G. Sharma and P. Key, Performance analysis of contention based medium access control protocols, in *Proceedings of the 25th Annual Joint Conference of the IEEE Computer and Communications Societies (INFOCOM)*, pp. 1–12, 2006.

[38] D. Gruhl, D. Liben-Nowell, R. V. Guha and A. Tomkins, Information diffusion through blogspace, in S. I. Feldman, M. Uretsky, M. Najork and C. E. Wills, editors, *Proceedings of the 13th International World Wide Web Conference*, pp. 491–501, ACM Press, 2004.

[39] L. Harper, Optimal assignment of numbers to vertices, *Journal of the Society for Industrial and Applied Mathematics*, **12**(1), 131–135, 1964.

[40] T. E. Harris, *The Theory of Branching Processes*, Dover, 1989.

[41] P. Jagers, *Branching Processes with Biological Applications*, Wiley, London, 1975.

[42] S. Janson, T. Luczak and A. Ruciński, *Random Graphs*, Wiley, 2000.

[43] M. Kearns, S. Surit and N. Monfort, An experimental study of the coloring problem on human subject networks, *Science*, **313**, 824–827, 2006.

[44] D. Kempe, J. Kleinberg and E. Tardos, Influential nodes in a diffusion model for social networks, in *International Colloquium on Automata, Languages and Programming (ICALP)*, pp. 1127–1138, 2005.

[45] W. O. Kermack and A. G. McKendrick, A contribution to the mathematical theory of epidemics, *Proceedings of the Royal Society of London, Series A*, **115**(772), 700–721, 1927.

[46] J. Kleinberg, The small-world phenomenon: an algorithmic perspective, in *Proceedings 32nd ACM Symposium on Theory of Computing*, pp. 163–170, 2000.

[47] J. Kleinberg, Complex networks and decentralized search algorithms, in *Proceedings of the International Congress of Mathematicians*, 2006.

[48] D. Kempe, J. Kleinberg and E. Tardos, Maximizing the spread of influence through a social network, in *Proceedings 9th ACM SIGKDD International Conference on Knowledge Discovery and Data Mining*, pp. 137–146, 2003.

[49] G. Kossinets, J. Kleinberg and D. Watts, The structure of information pathways in a social communication network, in *Proceedings 14th ACM SIGKDD International Conference on Knowledge Discovery and Data Mining*, 2008.

[50] S. Kumar and L. Massoulié, Integrating streaming and file-transfer Internet traffic: fluid and diffusion approximations, *Queueing Systems*, **55**(4), 195–205, 2007.

[51] E. Lebhar, A. Chaintreau and P. Fraigniaud, Networks become navigable as nodes move and forget, in *Proceedings of International Colloquium on Automata, Languages and Programming (ICALP)*, 2008.

[52] P. Duchon, N. Hanusse, E. Lebhar and N. Schabanel, Could any graph be turned into a small world?, in *Proceedings International Symposium on Distributed Computing (DISC)*, LNCS vol. 3724/2005, 511–513, 2005.

[53] E. Lebhar and N. Schabanel, Close to optimal decentralized routing in long-range contact networks, *Theoretical Computer Science special*, International Colloquium on Automata, Languages and Programming (ICALP) 2004, vol. 348, issue 2-3, 294–310, 2005.

[54] C. Lefevre and S. Utev, Poisson approximation for the final state of a generalized epidemic process, *Annals of Probability*, **23**(3), 1139–1162, 1995.

[55] J. Leskovec, L. Adamic and B. Huberman, The dynamics of viral marketing, in J. Feigenbaum, J. C.-I.Chuang and D. M. Pennock, editors, *Proceedings of the 7th ACM Conference on Electronic Commerce*, pp. 228–237, ACM Press, 2006.

[56] J. Leskovec, A. Singh and J. Kleinberg, Patterns of influence in a recommendation network, Lecture Notes in Computer Science, *Advances in Knowledge Discovery and Data Mining*, 380–389, Springer, 2006.

[57] T. M. Liggett, *Stochastic Interacting Systems: Contact, Voter and Exclusion Processes*, Springer, 1999.

[58] T. Lindvall, *Lectures on the Coupling Method*, Wiley, New York, 1992.

[59] L. Lovász and B. Szegedy. Limits of dense graph sequences, *Technical Report TR-2004-79, Microsoft Research*, 2004.

[60] L. Lovász and K. Vesztergombi, *Discrete Mathematics*, available at http://research.microsoft.com/users/lovasz/dmbook.ps

[61] V. Mahajan, E. Muller and F. M. Bass, New product diffusion models in marketing: a review and directions for research, *Journal of Marketing*, **54**(1), 1–26, 1990.

[62] B. Mandelbrot, Information theory and psycholinguistics: a theory of words frequencies, in P. Lazarsfeld and N. Henry, editors, *Readings in Mathematical Social Science*, MIT Press, 1966.

[63] A. Martin-Löf, Symmetric sampling procedures, general epidemic processes and their threshold limit theorems, *Journal of Applied Probability*, **23**(2), 265–282, 1986.

[64] L. Massoulié and M. Vojvonic, Coupon replication systems, *ACM SIGMETRICS Performance Evaluation Review*, **33**(1), 2–13, 2005.

[65] S. Milgram, The small world problem, *Psychology Today*, **1**(1), 61–67, 1967.

[66] M. Mitzenmacher, A brief history of generative models for power law and lognormal distributions, *Internet Mathematics*, **1**(2), 226–251, 2004.

[67] M. Mitzenmacher and E. Upfal, *Probability and Computing: Randomized Algorithms and Probabilistic Analysis*, Cambridge University Press, 2005.

[68] M. Molloy and B. A. Reed, A critical point for random graphs with a given degree sequence, *Random Structures and Algorithms* **6**, 161–180, 1995.

[69] M. Molloy and B. A. Reed, The size of the largest component of a random graph on a fixed degree sequence, *Combinatorics, Probability and Computing*, **7**, 295–306, 1998.

[70] E. Mossel, and S. Roch, On the submodularity of influence in social networks, in *Proceedings of the Thirty-Ninth Annual ACM Symposium on Theory of Computing (STOC)*, 128–134, 2007.

[71] R. Motwani and P. Raghavan, *Randomized Algorithms*, Cambridge University Press, 1995.

[72] A. Müller and D. Stoyan, *Comparison Methods for Stochastic Models and Risks*, Wiley, 2002.

[73] J. Mundinger and J.-Y. Le Boudec, Performance analysis of contention based medium access control protocols, *European Transactions on Telecommunications*, **16**(5), 375–384, 2005.

[74] A. Nachmias and Y. Peres, The critical random graph, with martingales, *Israel Journal of Mathematics*, to appear.

[75] G. Nemhauser and L. Wolsey. *Integer and Combinatorial Optimization*, Wiley, 1988.

[76] M. E. J. Newman, Power laws, Pareto distributions and Zipf's law, 2004, available at http://arxiv.org/abs/cond-mat/0412004

[77] B. Pittel, On Spreading a Rumor, *SIAM Journal on Applied Mathematics*, **47**(1), 213–223, 1987.

[78] E. Rogers, *Diffusion of Innovations*, Free Press, 4th edition, 1995.

[79] A. Shwartz and A. Weiss. *Large Deviations for Performance Analysis*, Taylor and Francis Ltd, 1995.

[80] T. Valente, *Network Models of the Diffusion of Innovations*, Hampton Press, 1995.

[81] V. Vazirani, *Approximation Algorithms*, Springer, 2003.

[82] D. Watts, *Small Worlds*, Wiley, 1999.

[83] N. Weaver, V. Paxson, S. Staniford and R. Cunningham, A taxonomy of computer worms, in *Workshop on Rapid Malcode (WORM)*, 2003.

[84] D. Williams, *Probability with Martingales*, Cambridge University Press, 1991.

[85] M. M. Williamson, Throttling viruses: restricting propagation to defeat malicious mobile code, in *ACSAC*, 2002.

[86] G. U. Yule, A mathematical theory of evolution based on the conclusions of Dr. J. C. Willis, *Philosophical Transactions of the Royal Society of London B*, **213**, 21–87, 1925.

Index